D1252949

Into the Lion's Den

COVID-19 Through the Eyes of an ICU nurse in NYC

Laura Luther
RN, BSN

Copyright © 2022 by Laura Luther. All rights reserved.

Library of Congress Cataloging-In-Publication Data
Into the Lion's Den / Laura Luther — 1st ed.
ISBN: 979-8-9859301-0-8
eISBN: 979-8-9859301-1-5
1. Memoir. 2.New York City. 3. COVID-19. 4. Nurse. 5. Pandemic.

Dedication

This book is dedicated to all the nurses who have fought, and are still fighting, COVID-19. For all the people who have left their loved ones, their lives, and their sanity to offer help in the epicenters of this pandemic. Who have protested lack of PPE and uncooperative citizens and begged people to wear masks and stay home. Every single one of them has a story similar to my own, and many of them have kept fighting long after I left the ring.

"Risk more than others think is safe.
Care more than others think is wise.
Dream more than others think is practical.
Expect more than others think is possible."
— Claude Bissell

"If you want to learn something about yourself,
do something that absolutely terrifies you."
— Selena Gomez

Disclaimer

While the stories in this book are true, they are told from my perspective and my memory alone. Any mistakes are my own. All names (of patients, co-workers, and hospitals) and patient room numbers have been changed to protect the privacy of those mentioned in this story. Some genders and specific details have been changed as well, to further protect their privacy.

Into the

Lion's Den

PREFACE

I'M LAUGHING RIGHT NOW AT that word: *preface*. I can't believe I'm writing one. I *hate* prefaces. I always read them *just in case* they contain information pertinent to the story, but they're almost always boring, and half the time they're irrelevant. Well, skip this one if you want to. I certainly won't judge you. But I thought it might be helpful to provide a short timeline of the craziness that was my life leading up to the 2020 COVID-19 pandemic.

On May 13, 2018, I graduated nursing school. I began work on night shift in an Intensive Care Unit (ICU). On February 9, 2019, my husband Jake proposed to me. When I called to tell my parents the good news, I was met on the other line by my frantic mom telling me that my 89-year-old dad had had a bad fall and she didn't know how to get him up. This was the first of many falls that year, four of which would land him in the hospital, and the last of which landed him in a memory care unit for Alzheimer's patients sometime near the first of May. On May 10, I experienced my first-ever panic attack. I was at work when it happened, and it was so bad my coworkers wheeled me down to the Emergency Department (ED), where I spent the next six hours recovering. I soon got a new job at a different hospital on day shift in their Medical and Surgical Intensive Care Units (MICU/SICU).

On June 3 (my twenty-fourth birthday) my maid of honor and one of my best friends, Brittany, gave me a blue merle mini Australian Shepherd puppy. I had *always* wanted that exact kind of dog. I had also always wanted to name her Elephant. I did, but we called her Ellie for short. The wedding was scheduled for September 7. We lost my dad on August 30. I spent my husband's birthday, October 13, in the ED with another panic attack. Two months after our honeymoon, on November 18, we also lost Ellie. I spent the next four months living in a fog, barely existing, trying to bring myself back to life with therapy, antidepressants, and nights out at bars. I was *just* starting to feel more like myself in February of 2020 when, in March, the entire world turned upside down.

I've heard it said that a writer is the sum of their experiences; I think the same can be said for nurses. These are mine.

EVERYTHING IS CHANGING

"WHAT'S THE CNO DOING DOWN here?" I ask Brad. It's 6 p.m. on a Friday. I've never seen the chief nursing officer on our unit, so her presence alone is strange, but to also see her and our entire management team here at 6 p.m. on a Friday? It's technically their weekend already.

"Who knows." Brad shrugs. "Maybe they're trying to devise a plan in case we get hit with a bunch of COVID patients or something. Hey, do you think now would be a good time to ask Leanne if we're allowed to keep used patient socks?!" I look over and he's holding up two of the yellow non-slip socks that we put in all of our patient rooms. We both double over laughing at his stupid joke and then go back to getting ready for shift change.

Ten minutes later I see our charge nurse, Courtney, zipping by. "Hey!" I say to her. "What's going on?"

She stops, hesitates. "I can't really say," she finally says.

"O.K. Is there anything I can help with?"

"No, but I'll let you know. Thanks." She hurries off. She looked stressed. The sinking feeling in the pit of my stomach that began to bubble when I first saw the CNO starts to return.

Five minutes later Jack comes up to me, his eyes wide. "We're getting our first COVID-positive patient," he whispers.

"What?! How do you know that?"

"Because it's going to be my patient." The flock of management whispering in the corner of our unit now makes perfect sense.

I help Jack and Courtney stock the patient's corner room. There's an ante room outside of it to store personal protective equipment (PPE). Inside the room is a negative pressure system meant to continuously suck particles out of the room. We have four of these pressure systems, and they were originally installed to protect healthcare staff from tuberculosis. Before COVID-19, tuberculosis was the only airborne-spreading disease that required an N95 mask or PAPR and a negative pressure air system to protect staff members from infection. Not anymore.

Jack and Courtney get into what looks like a spacesuit but is actually a Powered Air Purifying Respirator (PAPR), and next thing I know, the patient is being wheeled onto our unit. I jump into the nearest patient's room and throw my hand over my nose and mouth. In hindsight, I realize that did nothing to protect me, but in the moment I feel exposed and unsafe, and my hand is all I have available to me. Up until now I have been digging my nose in the sand and plugging my ears pretending that COVID-19 can't and won't ever be a problem that personally affects me. I am sad to say I have never been more wrong or oblivious about something in my entire life.

Jack comes out of the ante room, his eyes as wide as baseballs, furiously scrubbing bleach wipes up and down his arms. "Are you O.K.?" I ask him tentatively. He is very obviously *not* O.K., but I don't know what else to say, and I don't really want to go near him because I don't want exposure to COVID-19. He just shakes his head slowly as he continues to bleach off all of the skin cells on his arms. It is unsettling to see Jack look so terrified. He's got to be like 6'5", and he's a body builder. He is literally the strongest-looking man I know, and his many years of ICU nursing experience and amazing sense of humor are often a comfort to me when I'm having a stressful shift. If Jack is scared of COVID-19, everyone should be. *I'm so glad I have the next five days off.*

I beat Brad to our usual weekend bar: Mission Taco. For a bar that is often so full that Brad and I have to stand for an hour or so in order to get a table, it is eerily empty. There are maybe two people sitting at the actual bar, and only a third of the tables are occupied. I take a seat at the end of the bar, order a beer, and frantically begin googling "COVID-19 symptoms and transmission" and "COVID-19 Missouri." I come across a news clip describing the rapid spread of this virus throughout the U.S. and press the phone to my ear. I am terrified to realize I know next to nothing about a disease I am obviously going to have to help treat.

"What's with the face?" Brad asks, taking the seat next to me and ordering a beer.

"Oh, I was just listening to a thing about COVID. Can you believe this place?"

He takes a look around. "Yeah, I know. It's never this empty." He takes a sip then adds, "It's kind of nice."

I laugh. "Yeah, actually, it is."

"You know we're going to get it, right?" he asks me, smiling as he jokingly reaches over to touch my face.

"Cut it out!" I laugh, pushing his germy hands away. Inside I want to cry because I realize with horror that he's probably right. And all I really know about COVID-19 is that it's killed people.

We've just barely moved past the topic of COVID-19, and what it might mean for us and the hospital, when Brad sees one of the ICU physical therapists across the bar. "Hey," he says pointing, "isn't that Erica? I'm going to go say hi!"

"O.K."

After a few minutes he comes back over with her and her fiancé, who sits down on the other side of me. And just like that, we're talking about COVID again. According to Erica, a lot of the physical therapists that typically work in the ICU have already declared their refusal to work with COVID patients.

"They can do that?" I ask incredulously. *I sure as hell don't have that option.*

"Yeah, I guess so," she says. "But I kind of feel like it's part of our job."

"Yeah," I agree. "I don't like taking care of flu or *C. diff* patients, but that doesn't mean I don't have to."

"Exactly!"

Covid seems to be all we can talk about that night, and I drink more than I intended to, because I honestly don't know how else to cope with all of these overwhelming realizations.

The next five days that I had off were the last before COVID-19 took over my life. I really wish I could remember how I spent them—they seem so precious now—but I can't.

By the time I'm scheduled to work again, everything is different. Courtney and Renee, who usually take turns being the charge nurse of both the MICU and SICU, are now each in charge of a separate unit. The MICU has been turned into the unit for patients known or suspected to have COVID-19. The SICU has all of our other patients. I've been assigned to the

MICU, which is being led by Courtney. "Be careful about what you touch or lean against," she tells me as we walk towards that side of the unit, "we're periodically wiping things down with bleach. I've already ruined most of my scrubs."

I learn I have two rule-out patients, meaning we're waiting to get their test results back from the city's public health department (which is currently overseeing all testing). "How has it been?" I ask the night nurse I'm taking report from. "I've never been on this side before."

"Oh, it's not that bad," he tells me. "All of the PPE just becomes extremely tiresome after a while. The donning and the doffing . . . and the donning . . . and the doffing . . . you get the idea."

Unfortunately, I soon do. We are each provided with a PAPR hood, on which we are to write our names in sharpie. The hood connects to a belt that, when turned on, circulates air. This belt is to be worn over a protective gown, which is then topped off with gloves. Upon exiting a patient's room, we are to remove the PAPR and place it on one of two tables outside our patient's rooms, throw away the gown and gloves, and then wipe the entire PAPR with bleach wipes for at least three minutes. Then the bleach must dry for at least five minutes. The entire process of getting into and out of a room takes like ten minutes, which is kind of ridiculous for an environment where we are meant to respond quickly to very possible emergencies.

We are also given one pair of goggles each and told that if we have a rule-out or positive patient who is on five liters of oxygen or less, we just have to wear a gown, goggles, gloves, and a regular surgical mask. We are told that patients receiving six liters of oxygen or more are aerosolizing their COVID-19 particles into the room at a stronger and faster rate than those on five liters or less. Since there are only about ten PAPR belts for a unit with sixteen beds and multiple nurses, physicians, and respiratory therapists all needing to share the belts, we are encouraged to just wear a surgical mask with goggles when possible.

I find a few N95 masks in one of the ante rooms and start wearing one of these instead of surgical masks into my rooms.

"We're not supposed to be wearing those," Courtney scolds me. "Where did you even find it?"

"In the ante room where we used to keep them. And why not? I feel like this is going to protect me better than a surgical mask."

"Right, but you haven't been fit tested. And if that leaks, then particles are going to get in. It's better to just wear a surgical mask."

I'm skeptical, but I trust Courtney, so I do as she says. I have two non-ICU level rule-out patients, so I spend a lot of my shift helping Courtney re-organize things on the unit and coming up with new and better ways to take care of COVID patients without adding work or exposure for us. We label the tables for the PAPRs outside the patient rooms with signs that say "dirty" and "clean," hang hooks on all the patient doors for our goggles, and continually stock the PPE carts with masks, gowns, and gloves. We work to decide which supplies are absolutely vital to have in a COVID patient's room, and how much of each supply we need. When a patient leaves a room, we have to throw everything away, and we are now beginning to worry about hospital resources, so we want to cut down on waste.

I appreciate the work. It is a good distraction from the thought that I might catch COVID and die. The day as a whole is still fairly stressful. Everything is so different, and it feels like we are changing rules and policies every hour. Cleaning staff are refusing to come onto our unit, so their job requirements are added to ours. It's exhausting to constantly be wiping down surfaces and equipment with bleach, and it takes forever to break down a room after a patient receives a negative test result and gets transferred off the unit. Nurses in patient rooms communicate with nurses outside them by writing on the glass doors of the rooms to ask for supplies they forgot to bring with them or for medications they need. It is both strange and exhausting to be limited in our ability to readily go into and out of our patient's rooms. We are used to popping in and out all day. Now we are encouraged to do as much as we can in a thirty-minute period and then stay out for as long as we can, until the patient's next medication is due, to decrease our exposure time. There's a chance that the more often we are exposed to the virus, the higher our viral load will be, and the harder it will be to save us if we actually do get sick.

When I ask my friend Erica if she needs any help, she thrusts a handful of medications towards me before even telling me what they're for.

"Yes. Thank you. *Ugh*! I can't get the family for my patient in seventeen to leave me alone. They call so frequently that nothing's even changed with the guy before they call me again, and then they're upset that I haven't done anything since our last phone call but I don't know how they expect me to get anything done when I've spent all day talking to them. It's ridiculous!"

Our no-visitors policy is new with COVID. While it's nice to not have family members physically in the way, several nurses are now dealing with what Erica is dealing with: because the family can't be there to see things for themselves, they call non-stop to try to get updates. Some families are more respectful of our requests for boundaries and limited calls than others.

"Meanwhile, my patient in sixteen is literally dying. I've spent all morning on the phone with her physicians to get orders for comfort care. I finally have them. I feel horrible saying this, but I literally don't have a choice. Can you go sit in there with her while she dies? And give her these comfort medications if you think she needs them?"

Her phone starts to ring.

"Ugh! It's seventeen's family *again*. I have to get started on implementing all of his orders before I end up putting both of my patients in body bags today. Can you do this for me? I'm so sorry to dump that on you."

"Sure, don't worry about it, Erica."

"Thank you, love, you're a lifesaver!" she says before picking up her phone to tell the family that yes, she's headed into his room right now and she'll give them a call as soon as she speaks to his physician.

This is wild. Normally a patient who is dying takes precedence, even if they're dying because the family and medical team have all come to the conclusion that treatments aren't working and it's time to stop them. And it's normally a big to-do. We let the family break the two-visitor minimum and bring as many friends or family members as they want. We order a comfort cart from the kitchen so they have drinks and snacks while they're spending the patient's final few hours on earth with them. We give medications to ease any pain or discomfort the patient may be feeling after we take their breathing tube out and turn off any IV drips we were using to keep them alive. I'm going to be the only person with Erica's patient when she dies, and I don't even know her name.

I gown up and enter her room. Check her wristband. *Cheryl*.

"I'm so sorry, Cheryl. You deserve better."

I look around her room. Empty aside from the breathing machine and other various supplies. And now, me. I draw up and administer the medications Erica gave me. Then I unplug her ventilator. Turn off her IV pumps. Go to hold her hand.

"It's O.K., Cheryl. It's O.K. You're not alone. I'm here with you. And your family, they love you, O.K.? They are so, so sorry that they can't be here with you right now, but they love you and they understand. They understand that it's time for you to go, and they're going to be O.K., Cheryl. They don't want you to be in pain anymore. You can let go. It's time."

Cheryl does nothing. I sit and hold her hand for a little while. I don't even feel sad. I just feel weird about the fact that the only person here to help her die doesn't know a thing about her. I don't know who she is, why she's sick, who her family is, or how many people her family consists of. I may not know who she is, but Cheryl deserves better than that. We all do.

A respiratory therapist comes in and starts cleaning up the room, as if Cheryl isn't laying there dying. As if I'm not sitting there with her as she breathes her final breaths.

"Umm, excuse me. But what are you doing?" I ask her. It's not a respiratory therapist I'm used to working with, so I don't know her name or why she's in this room right now.

"I was told we need this ventilator and this room as soon as possible for a new admission in the ED My boss told me to start collecting all of the ventilation supplies as soon as you guys turned it off so we can give it to the next patient."

I can't believe what I'm hearing. The *next* patient? This one isn't even dead yet.

"It's fucked up, isn't it?" She tells me.

Yes it is. Yes. It. Is.

"Are you willing to do this again tomorrow, Laura?" Courtney asks me towards the end of my shift.

"You bet." I tell her. I'm in it now. Nothing to do but keep going.

When I get home that evening, my husband won't touch me or let me past our doorway. "O.K.," he says, "you strip right there, and then I'll go turn on the shower, so you don't have to touch the door or the handle."

O.K., seems reasonable, I think. When I get out of the shower, I go to give him a kiss and he jumps up like I'm a zombie coming to eat him. "What are you doing?" he asks me.

I laugh nervously, I don't understand what's going on. "I'm trying to say hello to my husband. What are *you* doing?"

"I'm trying not to get COVID!"

"I'm sorry, *what*?" I can't believe what I'm hearing and seeing. My husband is standing across our apartment, looking at me as if I were pointing a gun at him.

"You know . . ." he says, starting to sound exasperated, "social distancing!"

"Yeah, in public. Not from people you live with!"

"Well, I think it should apply to households when one of them is being directly exposed to COVID every time she goes to work."

"And how exactly is that supposed to work, *huh*?" I'm getting heated. Everything today has been a lot, and this, this is just too much. "How is that supposed to work when we use the same kitchen, shower, bed, and couch? Our couch is not six feet wide and neither is our bed."

"Well I was thinking I could sleep in the spare room on the air mattress . . ."

"*What?* For how long?" I feel like I am being abandoned. The only thing that got me through this terribly weird day was the thought of curling up safely next to my husband when I got home, and now he's not even going to sleep in the same room as me?

"Well—I don't know, as long as you're caring for COVID patients I guess."

"That could be *months*. You really expect us to make it with you basically not seeing me for *months*? We've barely been married half a year! Are you going to stop having sex with me too?"

"Well, yeah. It's not safe."

I can't believe what I'm hearing. I can't imagine living in the same home as my husband but actively trying to avoid seeing him. I thought we were one of those "if you die, I die" sort of couples, and now I feel like he's saying it's O.K. for me to die but not him. We've been struggling to feel like "us" lately after losing our puppy, Ellie, less than two months after I lost my Dad. Things with us have just started to feel normal again, and this is definitely going to ruin it. I have barely been holding on by a thread since experiencing those loses, and he is a big tether in that thread. Without him, I'm afraid I'll unravel completely. I'm unravelling a little bit now seeing the terror and anxiety in the eyes of the man I look towards to keep everything in our lives safe and held together.

"If you want to sleep in a different room," I say, "you might as well move out, because I don't know how that's actually going to protect you. We will still be touching the same surfaces and breathing the same air. Households are meant to quarantine from the rest of society, not from each other. I am very careful at work. I have protection, and I haven't even cared for a patient who's tested positive for COVID yet. They were just rule outs. I don't want this virus any more than you do, but if I get it, chances are you will too as long as we're living under the same roof. Chances are also that we will be fine. We're young and healthy, and so far it's mostly just killing old people with comorbidities." I'm not sure which of us I'm trying to convince with my argument. "You knew I worked with sick people when you married me. There have been tons of days where I cared for flu patients, or *C. diff* patients, or patients with MRSA, and you still shared a bed with me when I got home those nights. I don't see how this is any different."

"People are dying from this."

"People die from those other diseases, too. All the time!"

"Yes, but *healthy* people are dying from this. People like you and me. Me especially. I'm thirty-eight!"

"Exactly, Jake. You're thirty-eight. You're not in your fifties. You don't have any diseases or medical conditions. You should be fine!"

"But that doesn't mean I will be. Why do you want to risk my life?"

I'm feeling exasperated now. "Because I have to risk *my* life! Because I can't do my job if I let myself think like you. Do you understand that? *I can't do my job if I let myself think that way.* And I *have* to do my job."

"No, you don't. Just quit! We'll be fine."

"Are you kidding me? We don't even share a bank account, which is something *you* want by the way, and you want me to quit my job and live off of your income? When you're not even going to work right now *because the world has shut down*?

Jake, I can't quit. *This is my job.* I signed up to care for sick people. And when you married me, you signed up for it too."

"I honestly don't know why I married a nurse," he says more to himself than to me. "I'm the biggest germaphobe I know."

"Wow Jake. Nice. Thanks for that. No 'Wow, babe, I'm so proud of you for risking your life to save strangers.' No 'How was your day, honey?' Which was VERY FUCKING STRESSFUL thank you for asking. Just 'I don't know why I let myself marry a nurse.' Cool. Awesome. Well, if you sleep on that air mattress tonight you better start looking for a new apartment tomorrow, because I'm not willing to be my husband's roommate. Sorry."

With that, I slam our bedroom door and get ready for bed. After all, I have to work tomorrow. Taking care of sick people. Jake has always stressed that his job as an attorney is both more important and more stressful than mine, but I'll be damned if he entertains that idea for even a second in the midst of a pandemic. Perhaps I'm being selfish in insisting that Jake "expose" himself to me, but I've lost enough normalcy for one day. And as I'll soon learn, that normalcy isn't coming back anytime soon. And I'm about to lose a lot more.

Later, I feel Jake get into bed beside me. *Good choice*, I think, and I roll away from him to rest up for another day.

TIME'S UP FOR TOM

THE NEXT DAY AT WORK I have my two non-ICU rule-out patients back, so I continue to help Courtney with the organizing and stocking of the unit. I'm walking around filling PPE carts with gowns when my manager tells me not to do that anymore.

"Oh, O.K. Why not?"

"We've been told to collect all of the PPE and take it to a central location in the hospital."

"But we're using it," I say.

"I know, but our hospital is running low on gowns and masks, so I'm supposed to collect all the extras we have stocked and take them to central supply." With that, she goes around and takes all the boxes of masks and gowns that I've added to the PPE carts off the unit. We are barely left with enough to get through one shift.

The following day we are told that we get one paper gown per shift per patient room. We are to hang it on the patient's door when we are done so other staff members, such as physicians and respiratory therapists, can use them too. We are each given one surgical mask, which we're expected to make last an entire shift, even though they, along with the gowns, are designed for single use only. There was once a time where I would have been yelled at for using either item more than once in a five-minute period if, during that five minutes, I exited and re-entered a patient's room. Now they want us to make them last for nearly thirteen hours? We might as well just stop wearing them.

I won't lie: as much as this new policy is bullshit and totally unsafe and unfair for us, it's kind of fun to watch physicians freak out about it. The looks on some of their faces when we tell them there is one gown per patient for *everyone* to use is just priceless. *Welcome to our world*. My friend Mike starts calling the MICU the RICU (for Rona ICU, obviously) and it sticks. Courtney is eternally in charge of that unit, and she starts trying to assign nurses who tell her they're O.K. with working there, which means we all get used to being there every shift and having policies change, change again, change back, and then change yet again nearly every hour of every day.

One day the policy is that if we have a code, we're going to take the entire crash cart into the patient's room, the next day we're just going to take the top two drawers, so we contaminate fewer supplies. Before this can even get put into practice the medical director decides this is a safety risk and we are going to go back to taking the entire cart in. One moment we're re-using isolation gowns, the next moment we're wearing chemo gowns instead. One day, rule-out patients can't be assigned with other rule-out patients, the next day that's no longer a possibility and therefore no longer a concern. Sometimes it takes five days to receive COVID test results, sometimes only two. First, we're only supposed to wear our surgical masks when we're in a patient's room, then we're supposed to wear them all the time upon entering the hospital. It gets hard to keep up, and the ever-present smell of bleach that we incessantly wipe and re-wipe all the nursing station surfaces with probably starts to go to our heads.

At the end of the week, Courtney asks me whether I can pick up an extra shift. Normally, I would say no, since it would put me at four shifts in a row (nurses typically work only three twelve-hour shifts a week), but things are still a bit tense between Jake and me, and I cope best with stress by avoiding it with busy-ness, so I say yes. I've had my two non-ICU patients all week, so I've spent most of my time helping to implement the ever-changing policies and breaking down patient rooms after the patients are transferred, and then getting them ready for admissions once they're clean. Halfway through my fourth shift, one of my patients finally gets a negative test result and is promptly transferred off the unit, leaving me open for an admission. Around 4 p.m., I get one. Her name is Claire, and she is a known COVID positive patient.

One of the other hospitals is sending her to ours on fifteen liters of oxygen. This makes me very nervous, because all the other patients we've gotten on fifteen liters of oxygen have needed immediate intubation upon arrival to our unit. I scurry to get the room ready for such an emergency, but when Claire finally arrives, she has oxygen levels of 100%. Not only does she not need immediate intubation, she doesn't need the oxygen she is currently wearing. As it turns out, Claire had a panic attack when her provider called to tell her she tested positive for COVID-19, and the hospital that sent her to us was worried that her symptom of shortness of breath was COVID-related rather than anxiety-related. Per policy, the physicians plan to keep her overnight just in case, but they'll discharge her in the morning assuming she still doesn't require supplemental oxygen.

Claire is extremely kind and grateful for everything I do (and since she is young and in relatively good health aside from the COVID, I really don't have do much to take care of her). I've had panic attacks that have landed me in the ED, too, so I feel like I really understand what she is going through and the type of reassurance she needs to feel and hear. This has to be a scary experience for her. I, too, am scared, as this is my first face-to-face encounter with COVID-19. I remind myself that my patient needs me to be brave, so I am. There is no other option.

She asks if she can take a picture with me to send to her daughter. "You kind of look like an astronaut," Claire says, "and I think that image will help my daughter be able to laugh about this situation."

I hesitate. Although I don't mind, I also know I'm not supposed to allow photographs; they could lead to a HIPPA violation. I explain this to Claire.

"What if I took it on Snapchat?" she asks me with longing in her eyes.

"Yeah, O.K. But you have to promise not to post it on your story or on any other social media platform."

"I promise!"

I kind of wish it was appropriate to ask her to send me our selfie. I do look like an astronaut. And I know I will never forget her because this is the first time I am *knowingly* risking my own life to care for another's.

I'm finishing her admission charting when our charge nurse, Loraine, comes over and asks whether anyone would be willing to pick up a shift the next day, Sunday.

"Can I have my patient back?" I ask her.

"Of course!" she says.

Hmm. "Would you care if I wore a black scrub top? Picking up a shift would put me at six days in a row and I'll need my last clean navy blue top for Monday when management is here."

"Wear whatever you want! We really need the help."

"O.K.," I tell her. "I'll do it." The most shifts I have ever worked in a row is four, and that usually makes me want to die, but Claire is so sweet, and I can tell I am a calming presence for her anxiety. I kind of feel like she needs me. I wouldn't mind discharging her tomorrow, and if she ends up staying, I wouldn't mind that either. She looks relieved when I tell her I'll be back in the morning.

Sure enough, the next morning they want to discharge Claire. She is the only patient I'm assigned to take care of this morning. I start the discharge around 10 a.m., and Loraine tells me that once I have her out of here I can go home.

"What?" I say. I'm pissed. Waking up at 5 a.m. on my only day off in a stretch of six shifts just to go home four hours into it does *not* make the early wake-up call worth it. "I don't want to go home. I need the money, and I want to help."

"You can break down her room after she's gone, but if we still don't have an influx of admissions by then, I'm going to have to send you home."

Shortly after Claire is out the door, our manager (who usually doesn't work weekends) calls a meeting on the RICU side. "We have maintenance people coming this afternoon to convert the rest of our rooms on this side to negative-pressure rooms. I'm going to need all hands on deck moving patients that are currently in non-negative-pressure rooms into negative-pressure rooms so that the maintenance guys can get this done."

"That means I can stay, right?" I ask Loraine when our manager leaves. "I'd be happy to help!"

To my dismay, she says no, but I can still stay to break down Claire's room.

It takes me thirty minutes to bleach wipe the wheelchair. I have to make sure I wipe all the wheelchair's surfaces since COVID-19 is airborne and there could be particles on the wheels. I'm still breaking down the room when Loraine walks by.

"Hey," she says with a mischievous look on her face. "I need you to become very busy. There's an extremely sick patient in the ED. They suspect COVID. I'm assuming he's going to come here, and when he does, I'm going to need you to take him. So just find things to do so our manager doesn't tell you to go home. And get his room ready. I think they're preparing to intubate in the ED."

Yes. "Can do!" I say eagerly.

I quickly eat a power bar, and then I proceed to get the patient's room ready. I will later regret that I didn't just eat my lunch right then, because I won't end up getting a lunch break. I buzz around the unit asking if anyone needs help. I attend a short demonstration of the Lund University Cardiopulmonary Assist System, or LUCAS, machine run by our Medical Director of Critical Care. Within an hour of Loraine telling me she might need me to stay, my patient is brought in from the ED. He's intubated and unresponsive. They've had a hard time keeping him sedated without tanking his blood pressure, but I'm told that for the past half hour or so he's been adequately sedated and his BP has been normal. The ED nurse is gone before I can get his first set of vitals. His BP is 80/40. Not normal. Not good.

I can't leave the room without taking off the astronaut suit, sanitizing it, and re-applying it. This guy doesn't have that kind of time, so I have to rely on my co-workers to get me things I need, and I'm going to need a lot in a short amount of time. "Someone get me a bag of fluids, make some Levophed, and get me Emma. *Now*."

Emma is our pulmonary fellow. She and the pulmonary attending stay in the physician's office on our unit in case we need anything emergent. I need a central line, an ART line (an arterial line used for invasive blood pressure monitoring), and orders for pressers, and I need it all quickly. My next blood pressure reading drops ten points: 70/30. Not good.

Emma comes in with her space suit on and starts to ask me what's going on when she sees the blood pressure. "O.K. I need a central line setup and an ART line setup, and as soon as I get a line in let's get a new set of labs sent down on this guy. Put in an order for epi and Levo and get them hanging as soon as they get here."

I yell out my door for someone to grab all that stuff and put those orders in, and then Emma and I get to work on putting in the lines. Typically, when we get a new admission that's this sick, there's a flock of nurses coming into the room to provide assistance in stabilizing the patient. However, the rest of the patients on the unit are typically more stable than they currently are, and nurses aren't usually tied up in the hassle of spacesuit-wearing. Also, nurses with known positive patients aren't allowed to help me, because my patient is just a COVID rule-out. We don't want to risk exposing him to COVID-19 until we know he has it for sure. That means more than half of the nurses on our unit can't help me.

"What can I do?" Brad walks into my patient's room in a PAPR holding all the supplies Emma and I asked for. He tells us someone is on their way to pharmacy to get the epi.

"Prime a bag of fluids for me, then set up the ART line," Emma yells. Everything we say we have to shout over the noise of the air flowing through the PAPRs. It's both frustrating and exhausting, and the three of us often have to ask each other to repeat ourselves two or three times before we understand. Emma is finishing her assessment as Brad and I get to work priming IVs. I'm starting the Levophed as fast as I can.

"I don't think this guy has COVID," Emma says. "There's something wrong with his abdomen. Look." She presses into his stomach, which is bulging a little and does not appear to move inward like it should. "Did they get a scan of his abdomen when they got the CT of his chest?"

"Nope," I say.

"What the fuck? If they're there and it's a suspected COVID patient, just scan their whole body! People are going to start dying because doctors are going to cry COVID and miss other important diagnostic symptoms, like this man's abdomen. And now he's too unstable to take back to CT, so I have no idea what the problem there is. But if it's an internal bleed of some sort, that would explain why his blood pressure is dropping so quickly."

"Could he go to surgery even if that was the problem?" I ask her.

"No, he's too unstable. You're right. They wouldn't take him. But it still would've been nice to have that CT scan. Tell someone to order him a unit of blood. And hang more fluids. I'm almost positive his low blood pressure is a direct result of volume loss."

I spike a second bag of fluids as Brad finishes setting up the ART line and another nurse shows up with the bag of epi. I get it running as fast as I can; the Levo is already maxed out, and his blood pressure is not yet stable. Emma throws in a central line first so I have somewhere to put the pressers, then she gets the ART line. Thankfully, it's reading slightly higher than the external cuff presser was, which is common since it's a more accurate measuring device for blood pressure. I'm able to come down a bit on both pressers.

"Do you want me to start the propofol?" Brad asks Emma. She doesn't hear him. I start to say that he's just being an asshole—Brad and I often joke around at work and we obviously wouldn't want to give this guy anything that could drop his blood pressure, and any sedative will have that affect —but as he repeats himself I realize he's serious. The stress of the COVID, and this situation, is unreal. I start to worry that I'm not thinking straight either.

With the immediate threat seemingly gone, Emma leaves and Brad hangs the bag of blood someone's just brought us so I can actually do an assessment.

"Is it just me, or is his left side completely flaccid?" I ask Brad as I attempt to illicit a pain response on both sides again. I'm not wrong: his right arm and leg withdraw slightly from the sharp end of my scissors, but his left side has no reaction at all. "Fuck. On top of everything, I think he had a stroke. Should I even call a code stroke?"

"I would tell Emma," Brad replies, "but the only thing we can actually do for a code stroke is get a CT scan of his brain, and she just said he's too unstable to take back to CT."

I sigh. "That's what I was thinking."

We call for Emma, who confirms that we're right. A stroke is the least of his problems at the moment, and there's nothing we can do until we figure out what's causing his drop in blood pressure.

"Is there anything else I can do for you?" Brad asks me once the blood is running.

"No, I think I'm O.K. I'm going to try to chart my assessment in here just in case his pressers need a little more tweaking. Thank you so much. You're a life saver."

At this point I've turned off the epi and cut the amount of Levo in half. His blood pressure is tolerating it. The fluids are almost done infusing. I am trying to get an antibiotic the admitting doctor has ordered primed and hanging when I see his heart rate start to drop.

Fuck, he's going to code. I try to scramble to get the epi infusing again, but the IV pump is too slow. I don't have time. I am alone in this room. I need help, now. I hit the code button and start compressions. After about thirty compressions I am exhausted thanks to the weight of the PAPR and the heat caused by my protective gown. After a few minutes, I am still the only person in the room. I look to my left and it seems like the whole unit is just standing helplessly outside my room watching. I feel like a zoo animal stuck in a cage.

I lock eyes with another nurse, Clara, who's holding the automated external defibrillator machine and waiting for the physician next to her to finish putting on his protective gear so he can bring it into the room. Her eyes are as wide as mine, but she gives me a thumbs up and a big smile through the glass door. It's all she can do.

Eventually, a couple physicians come into my room. One of them takes over compressions and asks me what happened, but it's hard to explain it to him because I have to shout, and I'm exhausted and out of breath from the last few minutes of compressions I performed. Someone throws the LUCAS machine into my room and everyone outside my door is yelling at me to get it on my patient. I just learned how to operate it, but I missed the part where the physician showed everyone how to put it onto a patient. I open the container and the device looks foreign to me. Everyone is shouting instructions at once, and the physician performing compressions is yelling at me to get it on my patient. I'm exhausted and I feel frantic and like my brain is short-circuiting. I bet if I didn't have a PAPR on everyone would see smoke coming out of my ears.

The second physician and I manage to get the backboard of the LUCAS machine under the patient. By then, there's another nurse in my room, and she knows how to attach the top part. While she's doing that, I frantically program the IV pump to get the epi running again, and I change the dose of both the epi and the Levo to max. Blood is pooling in the bed near my patient's head and abdomen and we realize it's coming out of his OG—that is, orogastric, or mouth—tube and ART line site.

"He's in DIC," one of the doctors shouts over his PAPR. "Push fluids!" I'm scrambling to hang more fluids and push the blood in faster and blood is still pouring out of the bed and every time we do a pulse check there's no pulse and then after what feels like an eternity one of the physicians calls time of death and we stop and I'm panting and light-headed and my heart is racing and I don't know up from down and there's blood everywhere and the help is gone as soon as it came and my patient is dead.

I come out of the room. I feel defeated. I start taking my PAPR off for the first time in over three hours, and I shake my head and say "Fuck me" as Brad passes me to head into one of his patient's rooms.

I beeline for the bathroom. I need a minute alone. I need to breathe, but I can't breathe. *What the fuck was that?* I'm trying to process everything that just happened: My body acted almost on autopilot as I ran around my patient's room desperately trying to save his life. It was our unit's first COVID code. Because of the limited number of PAPRs we had been informed that code blues for COVID patients would be run by one to two physicians and two to three nurses. The LUCAS would always do the compressions, which would save resources and staff from getting tied up in the code. I learned this when I learned how to operate the LUCAS, nearly two hours before I had to live it out in practice.

I pull myself together enough to stop hyperventilating, and I reemerge from the bathroom. I walk over to my patient's room. It looks like a war zone. There's blood and trash everywhere—the results of our extensive efforts to save his life. His body is lying in the middle of it all. It's an overwhelming image.

Loraine walks up to me and I can tell she's been crying. "I've been with the family," she tells me, her voice cracking a little. "They are beside themselves. This is the hardest conversation I've ever had to have. I'm going to find a way to get them back here to see the body. Can you get the room cleaned up so it's presentable?"

"Yeah, O.K." I don't even know where to start. I have no idea how or why Loraine is going to get this man's family back here to see his body. We have a strict no-visitor policy in place for the entire hospital, and I'm fairly sure that the COVID unit is the place where this policy is and should be the strictest. *Their Dad/husband are dead,* I think. *They shouldn't have to die, too. It's not worth the risk. And why is she crying? She didn't have to watch this man die. She didn't just experience that code. If anyone should be crying right now, it's me!* It's an extremely unfair and selfish thought, but I have it anyway. "Overwhelmed" and "in shock" are understatements for how I'm feeling in this moment. I realize in all this chaos, I didn't even have the wherewithall to learn this man's name: Tom.

It takes me nearly two hours to clean the room and Tom's body. And it takes that long for Loraine to get approval for his family to come see his body. I have great anxieties about their coming back here. I know that if I am in shock, theirs must be ten times worse, and they're not going to care about the very real and life-threatening dangers of being exposed to COVID, because in the moment that's going to feel like the last thing that matters.

"I realize none of you are probably very worried or concerned with the dangers of catching COVID right now. In fact, that's probably the last thing on your minds. But it is a very real danger, and I would hate for any of you to have to suffer any more in the future, so I strongly advise you wear protective gear and wash your hands very extensively when you're done in the room." I tell them this as I take them back, two at a time, to see the dead body of their husband and father. Tom was only in his fifties. My heart is broken for this family.

They have to wear protective gloves, a gown, and a surgical mask in order to come onto the unit. The wife takes her gloves off so she can hold his hand, and touch his face. I understand her desire to touch him one last time, but I feel my heart pounding in my chest with worry as I watch her do it. I want to scream at her to stop, that it's not safe, but I've already warned her of the dangers this action could pose, and she's choosing to do it anyway. Further words would not make a difference. I take his wedding ring off and immerse it in bleach wipe solution for her. Technically, I'm supposed to give the ring to security and have them release it to her, but I can't imagine making her jump through those hoops.

Tom's family consists of his wife and three kids. The youngest kid appears to be high school age. The other two are older and married, and their wives are with them. One of the couples tells me they have toddlers at home, and they want to know what they should do to keep them safe now that they've possibly been exposed to COVID-19. I give them each a couple pairs of clean gloves and a plastic bag to dispose their hospital gloves into in the parking lot. I advise them to throw it away outside the building, to not take those things into their car. I advise the same of the surgical masks they have on. I give them each an extra gown, even though I know our supply is scarce. I tell them to put it on the seat of their car before they get in, to protect any COVID particles from getting on the interior. "Once you're home, strip as close to your front door as possible. Put those clothes in a plastic bag to keep them from touching anything else. Take a shower as soon as possible. Wash your hair and everything. Then we recommend you quarantine for two weeks. Don't go to stores, don't see your friends. Monitor your temperatures daily, and if you develop a fever or other COVID symptoms, such as shortness of breath, persistent cough, loss of taste or smell, or chills, seek medical attention as soon as possible."

They all nod. I appreciate that they are concerned about what I have to say; they ask good questions, and I am confident that everyone will remember my instructions. I'm impressed—I don't know if I'd have it in me to care if I were them. "I know sorry isn't a good enough word," I tell them, "but I truly am very sorry for your loss."

They thank me for taking care of Tom and for being a nurse in such trying times. I ask if there's anything else I can do for them. They say no. I tell them they're allowed to stay for as long as they'd like but they're also welcome to go at any time. Someone from the hospital will contact Tom's wife the next day to ask where she'd like to send her husband's body. I give her our hospital's main number just in case she thinks of any questions or concerns after they leave.

I'm nearly back to my patient's room when I feel my body turning around and rushing back towards the family. I sigh with relief when I open the door to the family room and see that they're all still there. "This might not make any difference to you all, but I lost my Dad late last year, and I think it would have helped me to know, if I hadn't been able to be with him when he passed, that he wasn't alone when he died. I promise you Tom was never alone. From the moment he arrived to our unit to the moment he breathed his last breath, I was by his side. I didn't leave his room once. He was never alone. I just thought you might like to know that." I don't know what's compelled me to turn around and say that, but I'm thankful I did. I hope it helps in some small way. It's the only comfort I have to offer.

Every face softens, and Tom's wife gets up to give me a hug and whisper thank you through her tears. I'm nearly crying myself now, but I feel it is not my place to do so; this is not my loss as much as it is theirs, and I don't want to take away from their need for comfort by creating a need of my own.

No one knows how we're supposed to do postmortem care for possible COVID-19 patients. It's almost 6 p.m., nearly three hours after my patient passed. I'm told I'm not supposed to touch the body yet, but someone will find out for me. I do the death paperwork, which often takes anywhere from thirty minutes to an hour, and call the Midwest Transplant Network to report the death. The MTN employee says she'll have to call me back because she's not sure what their policies are for suspected COVID-19 patients. Additionally, I was supposed to call within an hour of his passing, and she's not exactly sure how to proceed, since it's now been over three hours.

I tell Loraine that the MTN employee wants to speak with our charge nurse when she calls back. She looks at me in disbelief. "Why are you just now calling them?"

I want to punch her in the face. "Because it took me nearly two hours to clean his room by myself after we coded him, and you told me my top priority was to get his room and body ready for the family. Then once his family got here, you told me it was my job to supervise them as they viewed his body." I want to add, *I don't know when you think I would've had time to call MTN, not to mention I still haven't had a chance to emotionally regroup since losing* my *patient, so my mind isn't exactly in tip-top shape right now.* But I don't. I'm not O.K., and I know Loraine isn't either. As soon as I say what I do, her face softens and she tells me it's O.K. and that she understands, and she apologizes for not helping me make sure it got done. But she also says I should know that our hospital could lose its transplant accreditations if we don't call within an hour of patient expiration. Fortunately, MTN calls back to tell us they aren't even recording deaths suspected to have been caused by COVID-19, so they have no further questions. *Thank goodness, I guess.*

We are finally told that the only thing that we need to do differently for suspected COVID deaths is let the body sit in the room one hour before performing postmortem care, and then wipe the body bag down with bleach wipes once we're done. Tom's body has been in the room for over an hour, so it's time to do postmortem care. There's only ten minutes left in my shift; definitely not enough time. But Loraine doesn't offer to assign it to a night-shift nurse. I'm assuming we don't have enough, so I accept that I'll be here late and gather supplies to do it myself. Jamie and Brad are sitting next to each other, charting. They're my best hope for help. The rest of the staff here today is weekends-only so I'm not very good friends with any of them. I beg them both for help. Jamie has had our sickest COVID patient today and tells me she loves me, but this is the first chance she's had all day to chart, so she's already going to have to stay late. I understand; I haven't charted anything on my patient either. Brad agrees to help me.

We later learn from Tom's lab work that he had been in disseminated intravascular coagulation, a condition affecting the blood's ability to clot and stop bleeding. Many patients whose bodies enter DIC are unsavable because they bleed faster than we can replace their lost blood, and they aren't able to clot and stop their bleeding themselves. The blood that poured out of Tom's OG tube and line sites during his code makes much more sense with this knowledge. Emma's suspicion that he was bleeding internally into his abdomen is further confirmed by the petechiae (tiny round brown-purple spots under the skin, caused by internal bleeding) covering his backside when Brad and I turned him to get him into the body bag. It takes us forever to get his ART line and central line sites to stop bleeding once we remove them, and it's nearly half an hour past the end of our shift when we're done.

I thank Brad profusely for all of his help and go heat up my lunch, a sad microwaveable meal I grabbed from my freezer that morning. I don't even taste it. It's nearly 8 p.m. It takes me another hour and a half to do all of my charting, which seems silly and pointless since the patient is now expired, and at 9:11 p.m., I finally clock out. I've never had to stay this late at this facility. I'm exhausted. I still haven't emotionally processed the loss of my patient (something I think most, if not all, health care workers will tell you they take very personally), and even though it's the end of my fifth shift in a row, I am back for day six of six the next morning. What. A. Day.

NO TO NEURO

THE NEXT MORNING, I COME in emotionally hungover from the day before. I fully expect to see my name somewhere on the COVID side of the assignment sheet; that's where I've found it every shift since we made the MICU the RICU. To my surprise, it's not there. I scan the SICU side, it's not there either. *WTF? I know I work today.* I keep scanning the assignment sheet in disbelief. I finally find my name assigned to our hospital's neuroscience ICU. *Nope. Not today.*

I storm out of the huddle room to find our charge nurse. I find both Courtney and Renee on the RICU. "I'm not going to neuro," I tell them. I'm breathing heavily and I can feel that the expression on my face looks crazy and the tone of my voice matches. It's like I'm seeing and hearing myself, but at the same time it's not me. I am having an out-of-body experience, and whoever's left talking to Courtney and Renee is going rogue on me. "This is day six of six,"I explain "I just need to keep doing what I'm doing. I can't go to neuro. I'm basically on autopilot today, and I just need to keep doing what I've been doing. You have to send somebody else." We get lucky and another nurse volunteers to go to the neuro ICU, and I'm once again assigned to the RICU. *Thank God.*

Once my fate is sealed and I've calmed down, I realize how crazy I sound, and I apologize profusely to both Courtney and Renee.

"It's O.K.!" Renee tells me, "*I'm* sorry! I thought you might need a break and that neuro would be a good breather for you. I was trying to do you a favor."

"I see that now, and I truly appreciate the thought, but I can't work on neuro without thinking of my Dad. Working over there sometimes gives me PTSD from when he was in the hospital for his Alzheimer's, and I just don't have it in me today to go through that. I don't think I'm O.K. I'm sorry. I'll get it together." I realize as I'm saying this that it's true; I'm not O.K.

"It's all good!" Renee assures me. "I didn't know that about your Dad. I'm sorry. I'll keep it in mind in the future. Let me know if you need anything today, O.K.?"

"Thanks."

I'm assigned to care for two COVID rule-outs. One is what we call a walkie-talkie patient; alert and oriented, and able to perform tasks such as a trip to the bathroom independently. He's come to the ICU after an attempted suicide, so he's on constant observation, meaning a staff member must be with him at all times to ensure his personal safety. He's a COVID rule out because he's homeless, and we can't be too sure that he wasn't exposed to the virus under the bridge where he claims he and his girlfriend live. I chuckle at the fact that he insists that she's his "roommate."

My other patient is a woman in her upper sixties with cancer. They're fairly certain that her COVID test will come back positive, and indeed it does a couple shifts later. She caught the virus at church. She's currently requiring a lot of oxygen. So much so that per our current COVID protocols (if you can even call them that with how unofficial everything is), she should be intubated.

"She doesn't want to be intubated because of the cancer and her low chances of survival, but she doesn't want to be a DNR or comfort care either," the night shift nurse tells me.

"Why are they even allowing this?" I ask her. "We can't just say 'all COVID patient's requiring more than fifteen liters of oxygen get intubated' and then not make it true for the random patient that doesn't want that. Patients don't want all sorts of things. They don't understand the why behind 99% of what we do. She's either going to end up dying painfully from suffocation, or she's going to end up intubated. And by the looks of her current vitals, we're going to have to choose one of those options today." Her oxygen saturation is hanging out in the 80% to 90% range (normal is anything over 92%, and 100% is preferable), and according to her previous nurse, she's been like that all night.

"I know. It's super frustrating. I feel like doctors are always changing or bending the rules for random one-off situations, and then we nurses end up stuck between a rock and a hard place until nature forces an actual decision on everyone else."

"I mean, how low are they going to let her oxygen saturation get before they do something about it?"

"I'm not sure. My guess is it'll either need to sustain in the 80% range or persistently drop to the 70s before they'll intubate her. And just to warn you, she's call-light happy and kind of confused."

"I'll bet she is. She's probably becoming hypoxic." (This means there isn't enough oxygen being supplied to her brain, causing changes in mental status.)

No sooner is the warning out of her mouth than the call light comes on. I answer it from the nurse's station. "Hi, how can I help you?"

"I need some water!"

"O.K., I'll bring some in soon, in the next fifteen minutes or so, along with your morning meds." The call light rings three more times before I'm able to grab her some water and meds. During that time, my other patient decides to throw a fit over the fact that he's stuck in the ICU.

"I didn't try to kill myself!" he's screaming at the sitter when I enter his room. "And I don't have COVID! I don't have any symptoms. I don't need to be here. You don't need to have that spacesuit on to treat me."

I take a deep breath in my PAPR before yelling a response over its constant gush of air past my ears. "I understand that this is frustrating. And you're probably right, you probably don't have COVID. But we can't know that for sure until we get your test results back, and that takes a long time for everybody, not just you. Whether or not you currently have thoughts or desires to harm yourself, you told the ER nurse that you did when you were admitted. We take that very seriously here. Everything we are doing is to ensure your safety. Everything we're doing is for you."

"I can't stand it down here any longer. I want to take a shower. I want to get up and walk. And I want all of these damn cords off of me!" He starts to rip off his telemetry monitor and get out of bed.

"Woah, woah, woah! Slow down!" I yell as I gently redirect his actions with my hands. I don't have the patience or energy for this situation. I feel exhausted, like I'm arguing with an unruly toddler after being up all night with a sick, colicky baby.

"Listen to me," I say in what I like to think of as my mom voice. "I understand your complaints. I really do. But I don't make the rules here, I just have to follow them. And right now, the rules are that you have to stay in this room, with these monitors on, until we get your COVID results back. It's been five days. I'd be shocked if we don't have them back before the end of my shift at 7 p.m., O.K.? So, for the rest of this morning, at least, I need you to sit down and behave like the grown-ass man you clearly are. I will ask the doctor if we can change the frequency of your vital signs from every hour to every four so you don't have to be hooked up to quite so many wires, and I can get you an extra cup of coffee with breakfast when it comes"—he has been asking me for some since I first got here—"but that's about the extent of strings that I can pull. Do we have a deal?"

He seems slightly taken aback by my little speech. He fixes the monitor wires he has started to pull off and puts the leg that he has started to get out of bed with back under the covers. "Yes ma'am.," he says. "I'm sorry. I would appreciate that."

"O.K., great. As soon as I see the doctor, I'll ask him about the vitals, but I have no idea when he'll be by, so I can't exactly give you a time frame. Breakfast usually comes around 8:30, so I should have that for you in about thirty minutes. And as soon as I hear anything regarding your COVID results, I'll tell you."

"Thank you. Sorry to be such a pain."

"It's quite all right. Like I said, I understand your frustrations. I just can't do much about them."

It never ceases to amaze me that at the ripe young age of twenty-four I'm often baby-sitting people in their forties. I learned long ago that when they're acting the way that man just did, I have to verbally assert dominance, or I'll end up getting walked on for the remainder of the shift. I say a silent prayer that this will be his only outburst of the day. It's not even 8a.m.

"Room nine hit her call light twice while you were in there," one of the nurses tells me.

"Shocking," I say in response. "I'm heading there now."

I grab her pills and some water and start to gear up. She hits the call light again as I'm plugging in my PAPR. I roll my eyes. *You can see me. I'm clearly heading in there.* Before I can get my PAPR inflated all the way, she pulls off her oxygen, which drops her saturation level almost instantly. "NO!" I scream through the PAPR and the glass on her door. I rush in and fight to get the oxygen back in her nose.

"NO!" I scream again, in her face this time so I know she can hear me. "Kathy, you need this. You can't survive without it right now. You *have to* leave this on," I say as I succeed at pushing away her hands.

"No," she says half-heartedly. I can tell she's very weak. She's squirming her whole body in the bed, but it's not accomplishing anything.

"Sit still," I tell her. "Take some deep breaths. Come on. In through your nose, out through your mouth. Nice, deep breaths."

In all of her squirming her hair has fallen off her head, and I realize it's a wig. I chuckle. She's been here for several days now, and I'm not sure how the wig has managed to stay on this long. I remove it from the bed and put it in the closet along with her other belongings. Her real hair looks like peach fuzz, the tell-tale sign of a cancer patient who's recently been through chemo. *Why?* I think to myself. *Why would you go to church when there are so many warnings to avoid big crowds,* especially *for people like you.* It breaks my heart; this feels like it was avoidable.

When her oxygen saturation recovers, she finally simmers down, and I'm able to give her a few sips of water. She chokes on it. She's no longer mentally present enough to swallow correctly. I try to explain this to her, but I don't think it makes sense. I give her her IV medications and then leave the room. I need to speak to her doctor. We need to make a decision regarding intubation sooner rather than later. I don't even have the PAPR all the way off before she hits the call light again. I put it back on. I go into her room, turn off the call light, and ask what she needs.

"Can I have another blanket?" she asks me.

"Yes, one second." I yell out the door for someone to please grab me a warm blanket. I put it on her and ask if there's anything else I can do while I'm in here.

"No," she tells me.

But then it happens again: I've got the PAPR off and am cleaning it with bleach when her call light comes on. "Listen," I tell her, after pulling on someone else's clean, dry PAPR, "it takes me about fifteen minutes to get all of the protective gear that I have to wear on and off. You aren't my only patient to take care of. I can't keep coming immediately back in here after I've left; I won't be able to help anyone else."

"I just feel like no one's ever in here," she cries.

I sigh and soften my voice a little. I can tell that she's scared. "I know," I tell her, gently taking hold of her hand. "I know it's scary. And lonely. But there's a very good chance you have COVID, which means I have to wear all of this in order to come in here. I have to put it on to go into my other patient's room, too. It takes ten to fifteen minutes for me to take it all off and clean it, and another five to ten minutes to put it all back on. So, it takes me a long time to get into and out of rooms. All the other nurses have to do the same thing to see their patients, so we can't just run into and out of rooms like we used to be able to."

"But I'm *really* sick," she exclaims, as if she's an exception and I should be able to answer her every beck and call. "This is the ICU. I'm sick. Why are people not caring for me more often?"

"I know you're very sick. And this *is* the ICU. But you want know something?"

"What?"

"You're the healthiest sick person we have on this unit." Aside from my other patient, who isn't really an ICU patient but is stuck here anyway until those test results come back, this is a true statement. All the other patients on our unit are currently intubated.

"I am?" She asks me, wide-eyed. "Yes, you are. All the other patients have a tube in their throat to help them breathe. None of them are even awake enough to hit their call light. You're the only one on the unit who can do that. Most of the other patients are also requiring medications that need constant attention in order to keep their blood pressure stable. You just need this oxygen." I point towards the high-flow cannula in her nose.

"Oh." She seems unsure of what to say.

"I don't tell you this to make it sound like we don't care about you. We care about you very, very much, and I want you to feel like you're being cared for and taken care of while you're here. I tell you this so you can hopefully understand why people aren't in your room very often, O.K.? I promise to come in here every two hours at a minimum. I'll probably be in here more often than that. But I need for you to tell me everything you need for those two hours while I'm in here, so you can make it until the next time. I can't be answering your call light all day, or I'll never get to help my other patient. I care about him, too. I'm not telling you not to use your call light, but try to use it for emergencies, like being unable to breath or needing to use the restroom, and I'll address all other needs such as water and blankets when I come to check on you, O.K.? Does that make sense? Do you think you can do that for me?"

"O.K.," she says. "So you'll be back soon?"

"Yep, in two hours. And I'll call your room on the call light before I come in to make sure I'm bringing you everything you could possibly need before I do. There's someone watching your monitor the whole time, so we'll know if you need immediate medical attention. You're very safe here."

At this I *finally* leave her room. It's just after 9 a.m. *Shit*. I rush to grab my other patient's breakfast and two coffees, and his morning medications. I hope he won't be too upset by the delay. He isn't, but he does point it out. "You said breakfast would be here around 8:30 a.m.," he says with a smirk.

"I know. I'm sorry. I was with my other patient. She's a lot sicker than you, and she was having trouble breathing. I did the best I could."

"That's O.K., sweetheart, you remembered the extra coffee!" I'm amused by his change of demeanor since our previous encounter.

His sitter asks me if I can watch him for a while so she can take a morning break.

"Sure," I answer hesitantly. I'm not sure how long "a while" is, and I'm super behind already. I haven't charted a thing, and I need to talk to both of my patient's doctors regarding their plan of care for today. I'm also irritated that she's getting a morning break when I haven't even gotten a lunch break for the last two weeks. But I know it's her right, and I would need a break from sitting in a room with all the COVID gear on, too.

While she's gone and my patient eats his breakfast, I tidy up his room and bleach-wipe all its surfaces. At least I can check that off my to-do list. I still can't understand how the dirtiest unit in the entire hospital is now the only one that cleaning services won't clean. We don't have anything other than bleach wipes, so I can only imagine that the floor in here hasn't been cleaned since the patient was first admitted five days ago. It's sticky in some areas. The thought makes me gag a little.

Fifteen minutes pass, then twenty, then twenty-five. I stand by the door to my patient's room, watching for either of the physicians I need to speak to to come onto the unit. Since this became a COVID unit, it's even harder than usual to track physicians down or get them to come see the patients. It's like they're having a competition of who can spend the least amount of time on the unit. It's frustrating, because of all the patients in the hospital, these one's need the most attention, and the only ones giving it to them are us nurses. My charge nurse, Renee, sees me standing near the door and comes over to ask if I need anything.

"Well, I need to know where his sitter went. She asked if I would sit in here so she could take a morning break, but that was twenty-five minutes ago. I'm super behind, and I really need to talk to the physician for my other patient. I've been standing here in hopes of catching him if he comes onto the unit. The sitter isn't answering her phone, and I have no idea when she's planning on coming back."

"That's ridiculous," Renee says. "That's nearly a lunch break. It should count as her lunch break if she's really been gone that long."

"You're welcome to tell her that. Do you think you can find her?"

"I'll try. And if I can't, I'll contact her supervisor. Hang in there."

"Thanks."

It's nearly another ten minutes before the sitter finally returns. "Hey," she says in a chipper tone. "Sorry that took so long. I had to go talk to my manager."

"Uh-huh," I reply, tearing off my COVID gear before she's even in the room. "I have to check on my other patient. It's been too long." I hope she gets the passive-aggressive hint. I'm too tired to have it out with her. I peek in on Kathy. She seems to be asleep, and her oxygen saturation is holding in the low 90s. I page her doctor. I want to have a plan in place before she needs one.

Just as I finish leaving him a message, the doctor for the not-suicidal homeless guy comes by. "Hi," I say, stopping him from walking any further. "I was wondering if the patient in room seven could be downgraded to telemetry status? He'll have to stay down here until we get his COVID results back, but at least that way he could get a break from all the monitor cords, and then we'd know where to send him if his results come back negative. He's not requiring oxygen, and he claims he's not currently experiencing any suicidal ideation."

"I'll go see him, but I believe that would be fine. I'll let you know once I've made a decision."

"Thank you!"

The doctor soon approves the downgrade, and I bring in the good news along with the patient's lunch. "We can take off all the wires except the one monitoring your heart," I yell happily through my PAPR. It feels good to be able to follow through on even the smallest of promises/improvements.

Not long after his lunch, I am told by Courtney that his COVID test resulted negative, and we'll be moving him upstairs ASAP. I know he'll most likely go from a room on the telemetry floor to our psychiatric facility until the providers are sure he's not suicidal, but I leave out this unwelcome information when I share the good news with him.

"Thank you so, so much," he says. "I can't wait to take a real shower."

After he leaves, I begin the arduous task of cleaning his room. All the trash and linens must be taken out, the cabinets emptied, all surfaces and monitor wires doused with bleach wipes. Even though his COVID test was negative, we have to trash every single non-reusable, non-cleanable item that was brought into his room as a safety precaution for the next patient. I toss handfuls of empty, unused, unwrapped syringes. I throw out multiple empty canisters, un-opened tissue boxes, and unused gloves.

"There has to be a better way," I say to the empty room. If medical supplies for protection are so short, who's to say medical supplies for treatment won't become scarce as well?

When I'm finally done carrying all the trash and linen bags off the unit, I check on my other patient. She's still "resting." Chances are, she's become so hypoxic that her body no longer has energy to be restless. Her oxygen saturation is still in the low 90s. I leave her be.

My friend Erica comes over to ask whether I have time to assist with a COVID intubation. "There's a woman coming down on fifteen liters. Dr. A is going to intubate as soon as she gets here." "

"Let's fucking do it!" I tell her. I've taken to cursing a lot at work lately. I know it's unprofessional, but we no longer have visitors, and nearly every COVID patient is intubated and sedated. There's really no one here to complain about my use of foul language. Plus, I read once that curse words release endorphins, causing the human body to feel less pain. I am in extreme emotional pain, and I will take all the help I can get *thank you very fucking much.*

At this point, I am well-versed in the act of intubating a COVID patient. I gather all the supplies I know we'll need: an ART-line kit, a central line kit (the 18g for Dr. A), two suction kits, an OG tube, a foley catheter, a fresh gown and a package of warm bath wipes, wrist restraints (to keep her from pulling the breathing tube out), and a slew of tape, flushes, and syringes. I also pull the intubation box from the drug dispenser and draw up the various sedation and paralytic medications, carefully labeling each one. Then I grab my PAPR and put on a gown; they'll be here any minute, and we'll need to act fast.

The patient is wheeled in by two nurses dressed to the nine's in protective gear. One even has a hazmat suit on. I wonder how she got it; they haven't offered *us* any of those in the ICU. I settle the patient, hooking her up to our monitors, plugging the bed into the wall, and beginning to wipe her off with our antibacterial wipes, while Erica gets report from the patient's previous nurse.

Dr. A enters the room as I'm finishing the patient's antibacterial bath. "Hello Lawra," he says in his thick Middle Eastern accent, a name I've become quite fond of lately. Dr. A has been volunteering his time on our unit even when he's not assigned as our circulating attending. He knows we need the extra help, and he feels a sort of responsibility to these patients —as though a situation like this is exactly why he became a pulmonologist in the first place. I highly admire him for it. "Let's draw up ten of succs and forty of roc."

"Ten of succs and forty of roc," I confirm over our PAPRs.

"Is this IV good?" he asks me, pointing to the one in the patient's lower arm.

"I haven't had a chance to flush it yet," I tell him.

I grab a flush and quickly learn that the IV is, in fact, *not* good. We'll have to place another one, and quickly. We need it to administer the medications for intubation. I holler at Erica to grab IV supplies on her way into the room. The patient is very fidgety (a symptom that almost always goes hand-in-hand with lack of oxygenation), so I hold her arm still while Erica attempts to place a new IV. The patient looks terrified and is whimpering at the pain of the IV needle.

"I'm so sorry honey," Erica says as she fishes around the patient's vein with the IV catheter. After a couple tries, she tells Dr. A that she's unable to get the IV in. Patient's veins tend to deflate when they're this sick.

"I'll just place a central line. She's going to need it anyway, and she's currently saturating well on the fifteen liters. Lawra," he says, turning his attention to me, "can you please position the bedside table on the left side of the bed with a central line setup?"

"I'm on it!"

He then asks Erica to position herself on the right side of the bed where she can hold the patient still if need be. Since placement of a central line is a sterile procedure, physicians typically require at least one other person to place things on the sterile field and assist with any maneuvering of the patient or their supplies. At most hospitals, this role is typically fulfilled by an intern or a resident, but since we don't have those, it's always a nurse. I've helped with countless central line placements. Dr. A hardly has to ask for what he needs.

I'm thankful that I have the task of assisting Dr. A instead of holding the patient down. Erica is partially under the sterile field, PAPR hood and all, to get the patient's neck turned at the correct angle. The patient is scared and restless, and Erica is constantly cooing support and reassurance as she holds her in place. I don't think I have that kind of empathy and support in me right now.

"You're doing so good," Erica tells her. "I know it hurts, but just a little bit longer. He's almost done. You're doing a great job, just hang in there. I'm right here with you; you're not alone." This last sentiment is one that feels especially needed now that COVID has eradicated all visitors. The ICU is a scary place, and the choice between a breathing tube and death is hardly a choice.

Once the central line is placed, Dr. A explains what we're going to do next: "We will give you some medications to put you to sleep, and then we're going to place a breathing tube. We will continue to keep you sleepy once the breathing tube is in place. You won't be out completely, like you might be during a surgery, but you should be sleepy enough that you are unaware of any pain. We will place a catheter to drain your urine, and a tube to feed you. I can't say how long you will need to have the breathing tube. We will evaluate you every day and try to get it out as soon as possible. Do you understand?"

The patient nods nervously—small and slow movements of her head, up and down, barely noticeable. Erica promises to hold her hand and continues singing phrases of reassurance as Dr. A and I position the bed and the patient the way he needs them to get the breathing tube down her throat. I stand at the ready with the IV medications to first put her to sleep and then temporarily paralyze her to prevent her gag reflex from fighting the tube on its way down her throat and into her lungs. Intubation is considered an "aerosolizing procedure," meaning there's high amounts of infectious COVID particles released into the room as a result. We've limited the number of employees in here to just three, risking only the lives necessary to successfully complete the task.

"Thank you everyone for your help. You are greatly appreciated. Please stay safe," Dr. A says once we're done.

Erica and I stay behind after he leaves to place an OG tube and a foley catheter. We hang the medications Dr. A has ordered to keep the patient mildly sedated and comfortable. We clean up all the trash from the central line kit. We date all the new dressings so that future nurses will know when they need to be changed.

"Can I do anything else for you?" I ask Erica.

"No, I think I'm good. Thank you so much for your help."

"Sure thing, girl!"

I've barely opened the door to leave the room when Courtney runs up to me. "Hey," she says, sounding out of breath, "your patient has taken a turn for the worse. They're finally going to intubate. I've got all the supplies ready."

I glance at the clock: 6:15 p.m. There's barely an hour left to this exhausting shift, and intubation—accompanied by placement of a central line, foley catheter, and OG tube—is nearly a two-hour job. Not to mention everyone is busy at the end of their shift tying up loose ends and counting final intake and output numbers. Everything I just helped Erica with, I now have to do alone.

Dr. A has already left for the evening, so Dr. B will have to do the intubation. He's kind of a curmudgeonly man, and despite being an attending in an ICU, nothing he does ever has a sense of urgency. He also uses as little sedation for his intubations as possible, asking me to only give 20mg of etomidate with no paralyzing agent. Most physicians give at least 40mg of etomidate *in addition to* a paralytic. Poor Kathy chokes on the tube as he forces it down. I attempt to be comforting and consoling like Erica was for her patient, but I'm feeling very stressed, and I'm afraid I'm not helping very much (although let's face it, neither is her lack of sedation).

A sleeping beauty for most of the afternoon, Kathy is now turning into a silent hulk. She can't talk because of the tube, but she's thrashing about her bed with new vengeance. She keeps trying to yank the tube out of her mouth, and despite my best efforts to restrain her wrists far away from the tube, she will succeed if I physically release her wrists. Dr. B left the second his part of this job was done. I need a sedative. I need this woman to calm down so I can safely finish inserting all the other tubes that one is gifted along with a breathing tube.

I hit the room's call light to signal that I need help. A nurse runs up to the door and opens it just a crack to ask what I need. "I need orders for sedation. She won't calm down," I yell back. Then I snap at Kathy, "Leave that alone! You need this tube to breathe. Try to calm down honey. It's O.K. This tube is helping you breathe." The nurse leaves and Emma returns in her place. I'm thankful she's still here. "Hey," I holler at her, "I need some fucking meds!"

"Yikes, I can see that," she shouts back. "How much did Dr. B give to intubate?"

"Twenty of etomidate," I say, rolling my eyes. Emma mimics my eyes with her own.

"O.K., just give twenty more to get her to calm down, and I'll go try to sweet talk him into some propofol."

"God bless you," I tell her.

The etomidate does the trick. Once it kicks in, my patient stops fighting me mid-swing. I know the sedation won't last forever, and I say a silent prayer that Emma is able to get me that order for propofol before my patient wakes up. I tie her wrists to the sides of the bed as tight as I can. I take a look around the room. It's a mess. I try to ignore that as I place an OG tube and hook it up to suction. If I don't get that in while she's knocked out, it won't happen. I don't even want to think about the fact that I haven't charted anything on her since 11 a.m., and I'm going to have to record all of this once I'm done.

A nurse arrives at the door with a bottle of propofol. I could cry at the sight of it. I quickly hook it up; she's starting to stir. I give her a tiny bolus of it to get her to simmer back down. The nurse who gave me the propofol also gave me extension tubing so I could get the IV pole out into the hallway, a tactic we recently started using so that we're able to titrate medications at a moment's notice without having to gown up in protective gear and enter the patient's room.

As I hook the various extensions onto the primary tubing, I notice they're smaller than usual. I hit the call light. My friend Kristen walks over. "Hey babe, what do you need?" she asks, sliding the door open just enough to let sound enter through.

"What the fuck is this tubing? I need the MRI stuff. This looks like PCA extension."

"It is, but that's what we've been using. We're out of the MRI tubing."

"Fuck. Are you sure this is going to work? It's taking a million years to prime. I have little confidence that it's going to infuse properly."

"It's worked for me. Do you need anything else?"

"I'm going to need to place a Foley," I sigh.

"Just tell night shift you didn't have time. They can do it. We're all swamped right now."

"O.K., thanks."

I'm still trying to get the propofol to cooperate when Emma returns to my door. "Are you O.K.?" she shouts through the glass.

I look around at the mess, and then I draw an upside-down smiley face on the door.

She laughs. "I love you!" she says between snorts. But then she says, "uh-oh." She's looking at my monitor. My patient's blood pressure has dropped significantly since we last checked it. I press the button to retake her blood pressure. Emma and I both hold our breath and cross our fingers, willing the last number to have been a mistake. The new blood pressure is lower than the last.

"I'll have someone bring you Levo," Emma says. "Pause the propofol."

Damn it.

Within moments of pausing the propofol, my patient is once again attempting to remove her breathing tube.

"Try to relax," I shout at her through my PAPR. "You need this tube to breathe," I remind her. She either can't hear me, doesn't understand, or doesn't care. Her fights against the restraints and my efforts are ferocious.

Without the propofol, her blood pressure returns to an acceptable level before I have a chance to program an IV pump with Levo. I give her a small bump of propofol once I've finished priming all the extension tubing. I scan all of the medications, shove the IV pole out the door of the room, and then hastily clean it. There are about ten minutes left before night shift gets here. I feel bad; I'll be passing on a shit-show.

When I finally get to leave her room and take my PAPR off, it feels like taking a breath of air after breaking free from the grip of someone holding me underwater. I bump up the titrations of both the propofol and the Levo. Night shift can always try to wean her down from both, but they'll have a better start to their shift if she's well-sedated right now. I see the nurse who had her the night before at the nurse's station. I'm so relieved I don't have to explain all of this to someone new that I could cry.

"Rough day?" she asks, walking up to me as I finish dousing my PAPR with bleach.

"We both knew it would be," I reply.

"Looks like you talked them into intubating," she says with a nod towards our patient.

"Quite the opposite. As I predicted this morning"—which at this point feels like it was years ago—"they pussy-footed around until they had no choice but to make one for her. Of course, by that time the only person here was Dr. B."

She sighs in understanding.

"And everyone else was busy wrapping up their end-of-shift stuff," I continue. "I've had an impossible time getting her sedated. She responds really well to propofol, but it drops her pressures. I decided to just increase the dose of both her propofol and her Levo and let you figure it out. I'm sorry. And no one was able to help me place a Foley, so you'll have to do it. I managed to grab an OG tube, though," I offer.

"It's all good. I know how it is. Are they going to place a central line for the Levo?"

"Well, Dr. B left, so I don't know. Emma got me the order for the Levo, but she needs an attending to order us placement of a line."

"O.K., I'll see if one of the night shift docs will do it."

I grab a pack of antibacterial wipes and head to the locker room. I grab my lunch (now dinner—again) and throw it in the microwave. Then I strip out of surgical scrubs, wipe my arms and legs off with the antibacterial wipes, and change into my sweats, which I've started wearing into and out of the hospital in an attempt to keep COVID out of my car and home.

"What are you doing?" Kristin asks me as I pull my lunch-now-dinner out of the microwave.

"Well, I guess I'm eating my lunch for dinner as I chart on the shit-show of a shift I just had. I figured I might as well be comfortable while I do it."

"Man, that sucks. Hope you don't have to stay too late!"

I walk past a couple of physicians complaining that they shouldn't have to put in a central line. I can only assume they're talking about my patient. I roll my eyes.

It's irritating to me when people in healthcare can't just do their job. Yes, it sucks to have to do something that the previous shift couldn't get done. It sucks to have to stay late when there's an emergency with your patient. It sucks to get a new patient right after transferring a previous one. It sucks to have to clean up shit. It sucks to have to bathe and change the bedsheets of people who are 300 pounds. But it's our job. We knew it when we signed up for it. It's hard and taxing and exhausting, and sometimes it feels like no matter how hard we work we're still not doing enough. But it's our fucking job.

That said, I disagree with the notion that we signed up for the COVID pandemic. Let me be very clear when I say that this pandemic is *not* what we signed up for when we became healthcare professionals. Did we sign up to care for sick people with diseases that could possibly infect us? Did we sign up to have our hospitals full to the brim with sick patients? Did we sign up to witness death? Did we sign up to care for those affected by a pandemic, should one ever arise like it has now? Yes, yes, yes, and yes. But just like a soldier does not sign up to go to battle without camo and a gun, we did *not* sign up to do these things without proper protection.

We need—and deserve—protective masks, goggles, gowns, and gloves. We need more PAPRs than we have. Our patients need more ventilators than we have. Just a month ago, we were being scolded by our hospital's infectious disease coordinator for not immediately discarding a level three surgical mask after using it for a five minute task in a flu-positive patient's room, and now we're being told that there are no level three surgical masks available in the hospital, and if we should be so lucky to get our hands on a level three mask or an N95 mask, we are to wear it for the entirety of a twelve-hour shift. Someone please tell me why wearing the same level three mask for more than ten minutes when being exposed to the flu wasn't O.K. a week ago, but now it's acceptable against COVID-19, a disease we don't fully understand that has already killed thousands of people? It's *not* O.K.

In addition to lack of protective equipment, the hospital has decided to expose only "essential" employees. Cleaning crews don't enter COVID units. Nutrition services, including dietitians, don't enter COVID units. Lab technicians don't enter COVID units. Transporters don't transport COVID patients. Residents and students don't enter COVID units. Management certainly doesn't enter our unit. I haven't even seen the infectious disease coordinator. Physicians seem to spend less than five minutes on our unit. Even respiratory therapists are discouraged from spending large amounts of time on our unit. Nurses are now being trained how to maintain ventilators and when to change their settings so that we "no longer require this much help from respiratory services" to manage a respiratory disease.

How is it that nurses are the only truly essential medical providers? How is it that the healthcare system can be stripped down to *just* us? And why is it that we are not being compensated for this change?

Yes, I did sign up to care for sick patients in the event of a pandemic, but I did not sign up to be a nurse, a lab technician, a transporter, a cleaner, *and* a respiratory therapist. If you want me to work additional jobs, I expect to be paid for the additional work I'm doing. And I expect to be protected both physically and emotionally.

The only offer of emotional support we've received from management is a bowl of candy at the nurse's station (does that seem like a safe place to put it? At the nurse's station of a unit filled with patients suffering from an airborne disease?) with a sign on it stating:

> *We want to deeply thank and recognize the teams here for their unwavering response to the #COVID_19 pandemic. We see your hard work, courage, and commitment to care like family.*
>
> *– CEO*

I have so many questions, but the most pressing is: Um, why is COVID-19 a hashtag? Do you see it as a fad? Because we see it as a real fucking problem that you're doing absolutely nothing to help solve. Thanks, but no thanks, for the shitty-ass candy.

*****

I finish my charting as I rant to myself. I clock out after 9 p.m. for the second night in a row. I'm exhausted in ways I didn't know the human body could experience. I don't join Jake on the couch to watch TV or tell him about my day when I get home. He wouldn't understand anything I've experienced this week anyways. I'm even too tired to join him for a drink. After a hot shower I go straight to bed. The moment my head hits the pillow, I drift off to a deep sleep.

I wake up in a doctor's office. It looks to be outpatient. I am on a patient examination table wearing a mask and a patient gown. There's an IV in my left arm. Dr. B enters the room and tells me he's going to have to move me to a different room to begin the procedure.

"O.K.," I say hesitantly.

The room I am moved to is on the other side of the building. There's a large light over the table in the middle. Dr. B marks a spot on my abdomen. Then he removes my mask and replaces it with an oxygen mask. He's wearing a PAPR along with a protective gown and gloves. "Do I have COVID?" I ask him, but he seems not to hear me.

"I'm going to give you twenty of propofol and two of versed. You should fall asleep almost instantly."

I watch as he attempts to push propofol into my IV, but it gets stuck in the tubing. I realize it's PCA tubing. It's thinner than normal IV tubing, and the propofol isn't going in. I'm drowsy from the versed he gave me, but I'm not completely sedated. "Wait!" I try to scream through the haze of fog overcoming me. "I'm not asleep yet! The propofol isn't going in!" I can speak, but I can't move, and he seems again not to hear me.

He picks up a scalpel and then presses it down firm and sharp into my abdomen.

I'm screaming, but nobody is hearing me, and the propofol is still stuck in the IV tubing. "IT'S STILL STUCK IN THE —"

I sit straight up, breathing hard. It was just a nightmare.

Life these days is a never-ending nightmare.

I want so badly to wake up.

The next day, I'm assigned to care for Kathy again, along with a new patient named Lenn. I am told by the night shift nurse that Lenn was extubated yesterday only to be re-intubated an hour later, which has greatly reduced the doctors' original hopes of his recovery. His kidneys aren't doing great, so they're considering starting him on continuous veno-venous hemodialysis (CVVHD), but they want to give him twenty-four hours to re-stabilize after his re-intubation. When I talk to the nephrologist during rounds, he sounds like he's just waiting for Lenn's condition to head further south.

"I'm trying to get the family to understand that if we start him on CVVHD, the likelihood of him ever getting off of it, and that ventilator, are slim-to-none, so I just don't see any point in even starting it. Kathy, on the other hand, needs to be started on CVVHD this afternoon."

"Oh, really?" I'm surprised he wants to bother doing dialysis on an intubated COVID patient with stage IV cancer but not a twice-intubated COVID patient, but he's not wrong in saying that Kathy's renal compensation is much worse than Lenn's at the moment. CVVHD patients require one-to-one care, meaning they are that nurse's only patient.

You have to take a special class to learn how to trouble-shoot the dialysis machine. I've taken it twice since becoming a nurse, but I've never been given a CVVHD patient. Prior to COVID, it wasn't a very common thing we did. Now, half the patients on our unit are on CVVHD. With COVID, the first organs to start failing after the lungs fail are the kidneys, and patients who require a ventilator to breathe and IV medications to stabilize their blood pressure can't tolerate normal dialysis because it pulls one to two liters of fluid off the body in a matter of two to three hours. Someone who can't regulate their blood pressure without help from IV medications can't tolerate a fluid shift that big. The solution is to do continuous dialysis (CVVHD) to slowly remove one to two liters of fluid over the course of twenty-four hours.

I've been wanting to care for a CVVHD patient since I took the class on how to work the machine, and this looks like my opportunity. All of the other CVVHD nurses on our unit already have patients on CVVHD. I point this out to Emma, who's charging today. "Yeah, you're right. Erica should be downgrading a patient this afternoon, so once we get her patient off the unit we can give her Lenn and you can start CVVHD on Kathy. It'll probably take that long for the dialysis nurse to get it set up and ready to run, anyways."

I'm excited for the opportunity to care for a patient sick enough to require one-to-one care. I'm also excited to finally put what I've learned about CVVHD into practice. It's not necessarily difficult to do, since a dialysis nurse sets the machine up and can bail you out if you're unable to trouble-shoot an alarm. There's just a lot of hourly charting and monitoring of the patient's intake and output to ensure fluid is being pulled from their body at a tolerable pace for their unstable condition. Pre-COVID, one-to-one nurses would sit in the room with their patient for the entire duration of their shift, but since that would increase my exposure time, I sit in a chair just outside the room instead.

Although I would never wish for this many people to be this sick, the increased volume of high-acuity patients has quickly advanced my ICU skills, since I no longer have to fight the concept of seniority to be trusted with more complicated cases. It's the only upside of COVID that I've been able to find.

THE HANGOVER

THE FOLLOWING WEEKEND, Jake AND I are sitting on our patio having some beers when my friend Kourtney walks by with her dog (she lives in the same apartment complex as us). "Hey girl," I yell down. "How are you?"

"Good! Long time no see."

"I know Stupid COVID. Would you like to join us? I have wine."

"Oh my gosh, I'd love to. I haven't really hung out with anyone since quarantine was mandated."

"Neither have we, but I figure it's O.K., since we're both nurses and we'll be sitting outside."

"Let me take my dog home and I'll be right over."

Kourtney arrives shortly afterward, and despite knowing I had to work the following morning, we down a total of three bottles of wine between the two of us as Jake continues his drinking alone in front of the TV. I haven't been able to relax since my six-day stretch of shifts, and it feels so nice to get drunk and talk about boys and laugh at everything and nothing as if the world isn't falling apart around us.

*****

I wake at 4 a.m., nearly two hours before my alarm, feeling dizzy and nauseous. *Oh God, what have I done?*

I try to get comfortable enough to drift back to sleep, but every time I move, the world spins faster. I feel hot and clammy. I get up to look for the thermometer, but I can't find it. "Jake," I whispered as I gently shake his shoulder. "Jake, I'm sorry to wake you so early on the weekend, but where is the thermometer? I've look everywhere. I can't find it. I think I have a fever, and if I do, I can't go to work."

"O.K., gimme a minute. I'll find it," he slurs as he drags himself from sleep.

It takes a while but eventually we find it. I pray for a fever as I wait for the beeps to tell me the thermometer is ready to read, but it says my temperature is 98.1 F. "But I feel *horrible!*" I wail.

"You don't have COVID. You're hungover as fuck. Get up and go to work!" Jake yells at me as he falls over in a fit of hysterical laughter. He might still be drunk from last night.

Fuck. He's right.

I spend the entire morning willing the charge nurse to give me a reprieve from the PAPRs, convinced that the ever-present smell of bleach will make me vomit. I want to call in sick, but I know if I do there will be follow-up calls asking about my symptoms and reports will be made to God knows who about whether or not I have COVID. I can't call in, so I hope fervently for PAPR reprieve instead. My prayers are answered: When I show up, I find that I've been assigned to be a procedure nurse. Not only do I not have to wear a PAPR, but I won't be responsible for specific patients. I just have to be helpful to the other nurses. I might survive today after all.

My good luck continues as I circle around to ask the nurses how I can help. One of them asks me to run to the cafeteria to buy her an energy drink. While I'm there, I buy myself a large plate of sausage and biscuits with gravy. By the time I finish wolfing it down, I'm feeling much better. Definitely still hungover, but the urge to hurl up the entirety of my intestines is subsiding.

When I return to the unit, a nurse is getting an admission, so I go over to help settle her patient. The patient is young—only twenty-two years old—and already intubated. The doctors say they're certain she doesn't have COVID, so she's being admitted on our non-COVID side. This all happens before we are mandated to wear masks regardless of whether or not we are in a COVID patient's room. As we turn the patient to try to remove the dirty sheets out from under her and replace them with fresh ones, she wakes up and starts fighting to reach for her tube. We restart her sedation, but not before she thrashes hard enough to disconnect her ET tube from the ventilator and spray mucous on me and the nurse I'd bought the energy drink for. I feel my nausea returning. At least she doesn't have COVID.

Or so we thought. Shortly after we got her settled, our charge nurse, Loraine, comes over to inform me that she is going to have to pull me from being the procedure nurse so I can take care of the new patient; she's being transferred to the COVID side. The doctors are no longer confident in their original diagnosis.

"Are you *kidding me*? We've been in there without masks on! Her ET tube got disconnected when we were settling her. Her sputum was blown right in my face!"

"I know, and I'm so sorry. Make sure all of you write an incident report."

Yeah, because that's going to save me from COVID. Fuck. Well, I guess it's too late now. I know the situation isn't Loraine's fault, it's the doctors, but I'm still furious that it happened.

I get changed into surgical scrubs and geared up into a PAPR. "Sorry I couldn't keep you out of the RICU for long," Loraine says.

"Oh, it's totally fine. I'm just thankful that I got to eat some breakfast." And I mean it.

We wheel the patient over to the COVID unit. The only room available is back in the corner. As we're working to get her settled, her blood pressure starts tanking. I turn off her sedation and crank up the titration on her Levo, but it proves to be a temporary fix.

"I need the fellow," I shout to Loraine over the noise of the PAPR's air. My patient starts fighting to pull at her tube again, and it takes both my hands to restrain her, leaving me helpless to do anything else. "And an extra set of hands!"

Loraine leaves, and in her place another nurse, Karen, arrives, shortly followed by the pulmonology fellow, Tyler. Karen is immediately on my nerves, telling me what I need to do for my patient. "Titrate the Levo up and run the fluids wide open," she yells at me.

"Yeah, I know. But I can't do that and hold her down." Then, to my patient, I say, "Honey, you've *got* to relax. You're *very* sick. This tube is helping you breathe. If you pull it out, you could die." I don't want to scare her, but I need her to understand the severity of her current situation. I also need her to stop flailing her arms so I can practice medicine rather than wrestling.

"Titrate her Levo to forty and push two of versed to get her to calm down so we can get a central line placed," Tyler tells us. Karen pushes the versed as soon as I titrate the Levo.

I'm wary of titrating it that high—our protocol says the max value we can infuse is thirty, but a doctor is telling me to do it, so I'm hoping that makes it O.K. Tyler senses my uneasiness. "Forty of Levo won't hurt her. There's no difference between thirty and fifty at this point, but it can buy us time to set up other interventions for her blood pressure. Let's get a second fluid bolus dripping."

We don't have enough IV pumps on our unit to program that many drips, so we use ART line pressure bags to force fluid into her IVs as fast as possible. I manage to get two fluid boluses and a bag of epi hanging before my patient wakes up and begins thrashing around again. At this point, the pulmonology attending, Dr. G, is in the room. Frantic and easily frazzled, she is exactly the type of doctor you do *not* want around in the case of a crisis. She's also not a very hands-on doctor, and in this situation, she seems to think that helping to physically restrain my patient so that I am able to titrate her medications (something doctors don't know how to do, but probably should), is not part of her job description. I'm thankful for my hangover, because between Karen and Dr. G, my normal high-strung self would be hyperventilating and snapping at people by now if I only had the energy for it. My head feels clear, but my emotions feel stifled. It's the perfect combination for my current situation.

"Give her a bolus of propofol," Dr. G screams at me as Tyler and I are both fighting to hold down the patient's limbs, despite her having a blood pressure so low it would render some older adults nearly dead. "*Her blood pressure is fifty over twenty.*" I say too loudly. "I don't feel comfortable with that!" My stress has officially surpassed my hangover chill.

Tyler, the ever-calm presence, says that he'll push a small dose of propofol. My gut tells me it's the wrong call. But again, he's the doctor. It's on him.

The propofol instantly knocks my patient out while simultaneously bottoming her blood pressure, which I knew would happen. I titrate her Levo and her epi up past max.

"Give a small bolus of epi and then help me squeeze in another bag of fluids," Tyler tells me while Dr. G stands there with a panicked look on her face. I do as he says, quickly spiking another bag of fluids while Tyler physically twists the bag already hanging in his hands to force the fluid into her veins faster than the pressure bag could. Then, to Karen, he says, "Get a couple vials of bicarb and push those, too."

"Bicarb?" Dr. G asks. "But we don't know if she's acidotic or alkalotic."

"It can't hurt her, and it might help. The fluids are helping. We don't have time to diagnose her with lab work. We just need to keep doing things that are working. Once she's stable, we can figure out a more reasonable treatment regimen but for now, we do everything. She's only twenty-two years old."

The thought that COVID is causing all of this to happen to a patient who is younger than me is bone-chilling. I push it away. I have a job to do: save her life.

She responds remarkably well to the bicarb. We push a couple vials and a total of four liters of fluids before her blood pressure returns to a number that, although still abnormally low, indicates she's coming out of the woods. Dr. G says, "Good work everybody!" and leaves the room. Karen has been gone since she got the bicarb for us. Tyler stays until he's confident that the patient's blood pressure will stay where it is. I ask him whether I can have an order to give her more bicarb if her blood pressure were to suddenly tank again when he isn't around. He gives me a verbal order to give as much fluids and bicarb as I deem necessary throughout the shift, and to text him at the end of the day with how much I gave, and he'll put written orders for all of it in the patient's chart.

I make a list of the drips I have running on the glass doors of the room in dry erase marker. Every time I titrate one, I write the time and the new dose next to the name of the medication so I can properly chart it all later. This also allows physicians to see the numbers without having to interrupt what I'm doing to ask me. I've nearly finished tidying her room and hanging all the antibiotics the physicians wanted to start her on when Loraine comes to ask whether I wouldn't mind allowing my patient's mom to talk to her via our iPad.

"Sure," I say. "For a little while." I sigh. don't want her mom to be unable to see or talk to her, but I also don't want my patient, Imani, to get riled up again. I don't feel comfortable titrating her sedation much higher than it is, and neither she nor I can afford for her to pull that breathing tube out. I try to explain all of this to Imani's mom prior to turning the iPad towards her. I explain all the medications she's on, as well as the importance of the breathing tube. Despite my explanations, the mom spends the next ten minutes begging her baby to open her eyes. Which, of course, causes Imani to attempt to pull out her breathing tube.

I hold her hand down as her mom begs her to fight and keep her eyes open, but eventually Imani seems too agitated, and I kindly tell her worried mom that Imani needs to rest. I promise to call her at the end of my shift with an update, and I tell her that no news from us is good news. After we end the call, I have to increase all of Imani's medications again to get her properly and safely sedated.

I realize that it's nearly 4 p.m. and I have yet to leave this room since I entered it around 9 a.m. I call Loraine and ask whether she would be willing to stand in here while I use the restroom. I can't afford to leave Imani alone for that long. Her blood pressure hasn't been stable long enough to consider her in the clear, and if it were to tank as fast as it did earlier today, she'd be dead before anyone could get all their PPE on.

Loraine gasps when she enters the room. "Oh my gosh, I think your PAPR has deflated," she says, rushing over to me.

Fuck. All morning I've been pushing it up out of my face, but I haven't had time to mess with it, or figure out why it was causing me problems in the first place.

"Get out of here right now," Loraine orders me.

We both rush into the anteroom to get a better, safer look at my malfunctioning PAPR, but I can't help thinking *Too late now.* If the spray from my patient's ventilator didn't given me COVID this morning, this certainly will. Not only is this PAPR too big for my petite face, but the back has small holes caused by breakdown from the bleach wipes.

"Throw this hood away and find a smaller one when you come back," Loraine says. I nod wearily and then make a beeline for the bathroom. I really need to pee. And I'm thirsty. And hungry. And exhausted. This shift feels like it's lasted ten years at the very least. It hasn't even been ten hours. After diligently washing my hands and forearms for two or three minutes, I sit on the toilet, put my head between my over-scrubbed hands, and let out a long exhale. The "fresh air" of the bathroom feels as good to breathe in as that of a spring morning. I was in the malfunctioning PAPR without any breaks for over seven hours. My ears are still ringing from the constant outward push of air. My heart starts to slow for the first time all day. And God, it feels good to sit, even if only on a hospital toilet seat.

O.K., you can do this, I tell myself. *She just has to live for three more hours, and then someone else will be here to take over. You can keep her alive for that long.* I take one last deep, non-PAPR breath before leaving the bathroom. I hunt down a new, smaller, hole-free PAPR hood, and check my reflection in the glass door to ensure it's fully inflated prior to reentering my patient's room.

Loraine hugs me when I reenter. "You are truly a remarkable nurse," she says. "Great work this morning."

I beam back at her. Kinder compliments don't exist in the nursing world. I've been an ICU nurse for almost two years at this point, but I've been at this facility for only the last ten months. It has higher-acuity patients than my previous facility, and I typically get only the really sick patients, like this one, by accident (usually when I'm open to an admission, and the admission rolling in is super sick). I've been trying to prove myself with each super-critical patient, and it feels as though this is Loraine's way of telling me that I have. "Thank you. That really means a lot."

I spend the next two and a half hours trying to chart on the craziness that was this shift while occasionally titrating Imani's drips and making sure all the medications we gave her this morning got scanned under her chart in the computer. I turn her as gently as I can and brush her teeth and tube. I change her pillowcase, date her IV tubing and all the lines Tyler had placed that morning. I empty her catheter and put the total amount of urine she's produced that shift in her chart. Then I try to calculate all the fluids we've given her, plus the ones still dripping, and enter that total into her chart as well.

By the time I'm done with all of this, there are twenty minutes left before shift change. I'm finally confident her blood pressure isn't going to tank again. I clean my titrations off the door of her room before exiting. I take the PAPR helmet off, then the PAPR belt, then the chemo gown, and finally my gloves. I put on new gloves before wiping each item down with bleach. Then I go to the sink near the nurse's station and scrub my hands and forearms raw with surgical soap. I run to the break room to grab my lunch (a sad microwavable Lean Cuisine). I bring it to the unit's nutrition room, which just happens to be right outside my patient's room, and throw it in the microwave. I scarf it down from just outside her room in a matter of about three minutes, keeping an eye on her vital signs.

Once I'm done eating, I called Imani's mom like I earlier promised. I tell her that Imani is "critically stable," a term I like to use with family members to help them understand that their loved is stable, but only because of medical interventions. "Without the IV medications we have her on," I explain into the phone, "and the breathing tube, she wouldn't be alive right now. But she's doing much better than she was this morning, and hopefully that trend will continue throughout the night."

"God bless you. God bless you all for taking care of my baby," she cries. "I hate that I can't be there with her. Please let her know that momma loves her and is praying for her."

"I will, ma'am. Please know that I'm praying for her, too."

DO YOU WANT TO GO TO NEW YORK?

"DO YOU WANT TO GO to New York?" Brad says the minute he walks into the break room. "No," I snort, "not anytime soon. I don't have a death wish." Brad makes a face and keeps walking towards the locker room. Gina and I are sitting at the break table, putting on all of our protective gear. We've both changed into hospital-provided surgical scrubs and are now French braiding our hair so we can tuck the braids into surgical scrub caps to keep it safe from COVID-19 particles. The hospital has started encouraging us to wear the surgical scrubs so we don't have to take COVID-exposed clothes home. We wear sweats into and out of the hospital, something we'd already been doing when changing into our own personal scrubs, and the girls all wear surgical scrub caps to cover our hair. We've also transitioned from wearing only PAPRs to wearing N95 masks. I'm not sure if the hospital was just recently able to get some N95s in stock, or if the break-down of PAPR hoods (like the one I used last week that turned out to have holes in it) has led to this change in PPE. We have two break rooms now, too, one for the COVID nurses and one for the SICU nurses, so as not to contaminate their space with COVID.

"I've actually been thinking about taking a COVID contract somewhere," Gina says.

"Seriously?" I ask her. "Where do you want to go?"

"Wherever they're offering the most money."

"That's bound to be the worst spot," I tell her.

"Probably, but if they could make it worth my while financially, I'd consider it." She heads for the door. "It's not like they're making it worth my while here."

"True that." I plaster my N95 to my face and head towards the unit.

There's a sign that's been posted on our COVID-19 unit door for about a week that reads "district 9." It's the only sign that's been put up that makes me smile. Upon entering the COVID ICU, there are dozens of signs in bright, colorful letters that say things like "Positivity is power" and "You can do this!" *Bullshit. Let's see you fart rainbows and shit butterflies when you spend your day repeatedly exposed to death.*

I'm not sure who "you" is, but I'm assuming it's someone in upper management who made all these signs and thought they would do a lick of good.

Despite my annoyance with these signs, Lenn (the patient I had for half a shift a couple weeks ago who was re-intubated and the doctors were weary of starting CVVHD on) was extubated a couple days ago, and when I go to tell him goodbye and best wishes as he transfers out of our unit this morning (our first COVID-success story!), he tells me, "I just kept reading that sign outside my room: 'Don't give up.' And I told myself I wasn't allowed to give up. That I had to come off this ventilator and make it home to my wife." I'm glad to know these silly signs have helped someone. Lenn's goodbye warms my heart, and we're all thrilled to have our first COVID-positive patient make it off the vent and out of critical care.

I have fairly stable patients today, so once I've given them their morning medications, I begin making rounds on the unit to see if anyone else needs help. The turn of a patient here, a fetch for a supply there. The busier I stay, the less time I have to think about the fact that we all might be exposing ourselves to death. Courtney, our charge nurse, asks me whether I can help Brad set up a room for the admission he'll be getting.

I grab supplies and head into the room, where Brad is already setting up suction equipment for the patient's ventilator. "So," I ask him, half-joking, as I start to stock his cabinets with supplies, "are you going to New York now or something?"

"I think I am," he says, dead serious.

"Um, what? Do you want to die?"

"No," he says. "I want to make $65,000 in thirteen weeks."

"I'm sorry, *how much*?"

"Yeah." He smiles. "My roommate signed a contract last night. His recruiter asked if he knew anyone else who would be interested. He wants me to come with him. I think I'm going to do it."

"Wow," I say, "that is some serious money. That's like . . . what we make in a year!"

"I know."

"That would pay off all my credit cards," I start to marvel out loud, more to myself than to Brad.

"Yeah, I know."

"And my car . . ."

"So does that mean you want to go?"

"No, I can't. I'm married."

"I think if I were married and my wife said she wanted to travel for three months so she could make that much money, I'd let her go."

"You think that because you're not married," I tell him. His admission shows up and I help him settle the patient. That's the end of our conversation, but I can't stop going over numbers in my head.

My credit card debt is about $23,000. I owe about $8,000 on my car. That would still leave . . . like . . . $34,000! I wonder how cheap I could keep the cost of food. . . .

On my way home I decide I'll ask Jake what he thinks. *He'll say no and then I can stop thinking about this nonsense and get on with my life.* I tell him, tentatively, expecting him to beg me not to go.

"Well, if that's something you really want to do, I'm sure we could make it work."

I'm sorry, what?

"Yeah. I mean, I obviously don't want you to go. Thirteen weeks is a long time. But if it's something you really want to do, then I think you should do it. I've always regretted not joining the army after 9/11. This pandemic—especially in New York—is kind of like that for the medical field, and I don't want you to look back ten years from now filled with regret like I do."

"Wow. I wasn't expecting you to say that at all. Thank you. That's an incredibly selfless thing to say, Jake. Maybe I'll consider it some more."

"I think I'm going to go. I talked to a recruiter last night. They said as long as you have a year or more of ICU experience, you can go pretty much anywhere," Gina tells me a few days later.

So much for Brad's wish to go. He's had only about eight months of ICU experience. "Cool!" I say. "How did you manage to talk to a recruiter?"

"All I had to do was fill out an application with a travel agency, and within an hour one called me with potential options," Gina says as she changes into the hospital scrubs.

Huh, seems easy enough.

I haven't seriously looked into traveling since Jake said I could go. I think I was expecting him to make the decision for me, and now I'm trying to wrap my head around the fact that living and working in New York is an actual possibility. It's something I've always wanted to do: move far away from home, experience a new state, new scenery, new friends. Do something cool. Have an adventure.

Growing up, I dreamed of going away to college, the way kids always seem to do in movies and TV shows. Then, of course, I got to high school graduation and realized I hadn't applied anywhere. Nor did I have any idea how to. Even if I *had* applied to colleges, I wouldn't have been able to go away. My parents didn't have any money to spare, and I just flat-out didn't have any money at all. Not to mention that my Dad had a knee replacement surgery that year. It took a lot of rehab before he could walk on his own again, and my mom needed more help around the house than usual. I ended up going to community college and working full time at a Starbucks. I don't regret that decision. It kept me within a thirty-minute drive of my Dad, whose health gradually got worse as I worked my way through nursing school, and it led me to my husband. Jake came in every morning on his way to work for a venti iced coffee. Fast forward four years later: Jake is my husband and my Dad is dead.

Today is my first day assigned to the SICU since the MICU was re-purposed as our COVID-19 unit. I have the pleasure of caring for Imani, the twenty-two year old I saved on the COVID side last week. She is extubated now and waiting for a telemetry bed upstairs; she no longer requires intensive care. I don't usually enjoy caring for downgraded patients—they tend to be needy and time-consuming—but today I'm delighted to care for Imani. Not only is Imani not a needy, time-consuming patient, she is very much alive, breathing, and talking, a vast improvement from the last time I saw her. It's rewarding to see a clinical picture come full circle like this.

Imani is my only patient right now, which means I have a decent amount of downtime on my hands. I do rounds on the unit to offer help after passing morning meds like I always do, but there are only two other nurses on the SICU side; we just don't have as many non-COVID patients as we used to. I decide to use my downtime to apply for travel nursing.

That afternoon, just after I've finished submitting my application, my charge nurse, Loraine, calls to tell me I'll be getting two admissions.

"Two?" I ask her. "At the same time?"

"Yes," she says over the phone. "I'm really sorry, but you're the only nurse who doesn't have two patients, and I just got a bed upstairs for Imani, so you'll be open for two."

I sigh. "O.K." It's not like I have a choice.

The rest of my afternoon is crazy. My admissions come within thirty minutes of each other, and they're both actively unstable. The first patient, Frank, who's just been intubated, comes from the ED. I barely have him settled and hooked up to the monitor when my second admission, Larry, comes down. They had to call a rapid response on Larry upstairs. The nurse who gives me Larry's report knows next to nothing about him except that his blood pressure is dangerously low, and his lab work suggests internal bleeding. He needs a blood transfusion emergently, and none of the pre-bloodwork tasks have been completed, nor have the fifty other new orders his physician put in when they called the rapid.

Between giving blood and fluids to Larry to keep his blood pressure stable and unsuccessfully attempting to sedate Frank in the room next door, I feel ragged and worn by the end of my shift. And here I thought I was getting a well-earned break from the craziness of the COVID side.

I pull my phone out to play some music for my drive home and realize I have a new voicemail. It's from Michelle, a recruiter for a travel nurse company. She'd love to interview me at my earliest convenience. I call her back. I do the interview in the hospital parking lot. Gina's right. If I'm going to put up with this bullshit, I might as well get fairly compensated for it.

The next morning, I'm enjoying a cup of coffee on my balcony when I get a call from Michelle. "I got you a thirteen-week contract at New York Health System. Five-thousand-dollar gross income weekly for four shifts a week," she squeals.

"That's amazing!" I tell her.

"I know! I just sent you an email outlining the details. Could you pull it up and take a look at it? I want to know whether you have any questions before we proceed."

"Sure," I say as I pull it up on my phone. I skim the contract. "What does 11.5 N mean?" I ask. It is listed next to the word *shifts*.

"Eleven-point-five is the length of the shift, and N stands for 'nights,'" she answers.

"Oh. I don't do nights," I tell Michelle flatly.

"Oh." I can tell she hadn't planned for this. "Well that's all New York Health System has available."

"Well then I guess I won't be going."

Michelle tries to convince me consider it further since it's "only thirteen weeks." I tell her it's a strong no. I know from experience that it will be difficult for me to work four shifts a week even if I can get seven or eight hours of sleep after each one. I'm not about to risk my health further by cutting my sleep down to five or six hours a day. She offers day shift positions in other New York City burrows, such as Queens or the Bronx, but I tell her I'm really only interested in New York Health System. I know from idle research that its Manhattan facility is the only level-one trauma hospital in the city. If I can't work there, I'm going to stay at my level-one trauma facility in Kansas City.

Well, that decides that. I was unsure about the whole thing anyway. I tell Jake when I get home that if Michelle can get me a day shift position, I'll go, but if not, I'm staying at my current hospital.

That night, as my head hits the pillow, I look at Jake and think to myself, *I love this man so much. I'm kind of glad that didn't work out. I don't think I really wanted to go, anyway.*

LIFE IS A BLUR

THE NEXT MORNING, I GET another call from Michelle. "I had to pull a lot of strings, but I got you a day shift contract at New York Health System Hospital."

"Wow, really?"

"Yes, really! Do you want it? We need to act fast before another nurse gets it."

It isn't until the possibility is right in front of me that I realize just how badly I *do* want it. "Wow, O.K. Let me just talk to my husband one last time before we make it official, but I want it. I'll call you right back."

I go to Jake in our makeshift work-from-home office that we set up for him in our guest bedroom after his law firm made the decision to have everyone work remotely until further notice. "Hey, babe, do you have a second?"

"Sure, what's up?" he replies, still typing away at his computer.

"I need to ask you something." I think he can hear the caution in my voice.

"O.K. . . .," he says, getting up from his desk and following me to the living room.

"Michelle just called," I tell him after we sit down. "They have a day-shift position at New York Health System."

"Wow," he says.

"I want to take it."

Tears well up in his eyes. I'm touched. Jake does not easily become emotional.

"Awe, don't cry. I don't have to go!"

"You're smiling," he says, laughing. "I can tell you really want this. I'll be O.K. You should do it."

"Really?" I ask him, still unsure whether I'm making the right call.

"Yes babe. Really."

"I'm going to New York," I say tentatively.

"You're going to New York," Jake exclaims as enthusiastically as he can.

Jake goes back to work, and I call Michelle back. "I want it."

She's thrilled. "Oh Laura, you won't regret it."

I'm not entirely sure why, but I believe her. I agree to a verbal contract, and shortly after, I am signing a digital one online.

Later that day, I draft a resignation letter to my current manager. I debate strongly whether it's best to send an email or have a conversation with her, but in the end, I decide to do both, like I had at my previous job, so that I have my notice of resignation in writing.

"Once I hit send, there's no turning back" I say, eying Jake nervously. I still can't believe this is happening.

"Do it," he tells me.

I hit send.

The morning of my next shift, I am braced to talk about my resignation with my manager. I sent the email on a Saturday, and today is Monday, so I'm hoping she had time to react to it over the weekend, but I can't be certain because I never received a reply.

"Good morning!" I say cheerily as I step into her office.

"Hello," she replies, a little distracted.

"I was wondering if you had gotten my email this weekend . . . ?" I say.

Not looking up from whatever she's shuffling around on her desk, she answers, "Nope. I took an actual break from work this weekend. No emails, no calls, no work."

I can feel my heart rate rise instantly. "Oh," I say, not sure how to proceed. It seems like she is in a bad mood despite the "actual break from work" she says she had the past two days. "Well, I need to tell you something, then."

"O.K.," she says, still not looking at me.

"I want you to know that this is a really recent decision, which is why I originally emailed you about it, because I wanted you to know as soon as I did." I can tell I'm rambling, but I can't seem to stop myself. I'm not entirely sure what to say, and it's only 6:45 in the morning. My brain isn't awake yet, and it's becoming all too apparent that neither is my manager's. "Um, well, I'm not sure exactly how to say this, so I'll just get to the point. I've decided to take a travel position in New York."

She stops what she's doing and looks up at me for the first time since I walked into her office. She doesn't say anything, so I continue to ramble.

"I really appreciate everything you've done for me since I've been here, and I've learned so much. But my husband and I have decided that this is what I need to do." I got that "my husband and I" line from my mom. "Who can argue with you on that?" she'd said the night before on the phone. I hadn't been planning on using it, but in my uncertainty it just came out.

My manager takes a sharp inhale of air. "Well," she says tartly, "thanks for letting me know. What's your plan?"

"Um, well, my new position starts on April 17. I'm scheduled for PTO all next week for a race I was supposed to do in Florida, so since this Saturday's email was my two weeks' notice, that would make this Wednesday my last day."

She writes this down on a Post-it note and tells me I'd better go get report. I leave her office with an awkward "Thanks again, for everything." She doesn't respond.

That went pretty badly, I think. I knew from talking to several other nurses who were looking into traveling, Gina included, that if we wanted to take a travel contract we were going to have to quit. Gina eventually decided against the idea. She didn't like the possibility of being jobless when her contract ended. I don't like the possibility of it either, but I decide to panic about only one thing at a time.

I look around for Brad. I know he decided to take a contract too and was also planning to resign today. Even though he has less than a year of ICU experience, a New York hospital has decided to take him on as an ICU nurse if he is willing to work night shift. "I can do anything for thirteen weeks," he told me.

Selfishly, I'm hoping I beat him to the punch of handing in his resignation, although I would be shocked to hear that I have based on my manager's mood.

"Hey," I call when I see him. "How's it going?"

"Oh, fine," he says. He takes a sip of his coffee. "How are you?"

"I'm O.K. I just told our manager I quit."

"Oh shit, really? How'd it go?"

"Not well. She was in a terrible mood when I walked into her office, and I definitely made it worse."

"That sucks," he says. "Maybe I won't tell her about my contract today after all."

Yes, I told her first. "Yeah, you might want to consider sending an email or something. I basically just word-vomited until she strongly hinted I should leave her office and get to work."

The shifts that follow are a blur. I've asked Brad and Gina not to tell anyone I'm leaving. I know the news will be met with a myriad of questions and opinions from other people, and I don't want to hear them. I've just barely talked myself into doing this, and it's too late if someone manages to talk me out of it. On Tuesday I ask everyone whether they're back tomorrow. If the answer is no, I tell them my news so that I can say goodbye, but I ask them not to share it until I'm gone.

Wednesday is my last day, and I tell everyone. I'm so happy that this is the last time that I will have to come to work here that I don't care about everyone's opinions. I'm just ready to go. I give lots of hugs, trying to store them up for the lonely thirteen weeks ahead. I try to remember the face of each friend. I hope they will remember mine. I honestly do not know whether they will see me again.

At some point, Brad asks whether I can help him with something. His patient is sedated, so we chat while we change the sheets beneath him. "How does it feel to know you're never coming back here when you walk out in a few hours?" Brad asks me.

"Amazing," I tell him with a smile. He smiles back. We're quiet for a moment, and then his face turns serious.

"Are you scared, though?" he asks me.

"Of course," I answer, honestly.

"I am, too," he says.

"Well," I say, "it's too late to turn back now."

NO SLEEP TILL BROOKLYN

THE FOLLOWING TWO WEEKS FLY by. I spend a few days doing nothing—which I desperately need after all the overtime I've been working. Then I spend a few days hanging out with some friends from the hospital. They are excited for me and my new adventure. There are a couple of friends I see that aren't coworkers but are still nurses. Those of my friends who aren't nurses won't, and shouldn't, see me before I leave. I was taking care of COVID-positive patients up until my last shift. I am a potential exposure risk for everyone I see.

My mom says goodbye to me from inside her car, two parking spaces over from mine, in the lot outside my apartment. She takes a picture of me before we part ways. At the time, I just think it's a weird mom thing, but looking back on it, I'll wonder whether she thought that might be the last time she'd ever get to see me.

I pack three months' worth of toiletries (as if they won't sell those in New York) and approximately four outfits for each season. Although it's April, the weather has been hit or miss in Kansas City, and I've confirmed that New York has been no different.

Maddi, a former employee of the hospital I just quit, started her crisis contract a week ago at a hospital in Queens. She and I have been texting here and there ever since I saw her post about heading to New York on Facebook. I'm bummed we won't be at the same hospital, or even in the same borough, but I'm hoping we'll get to hang out on our days off. I don't know Maddi very well, since we didn't work on the same unit in Kansas City, but the few times I've talked to her, she seemed really nice, and it looks like she's going to be the closest thing I'll have to a girlfriend once I get to New York.

I weigh my luggage, repack, reweigh. I want to have only two suitcases since I'm going to have to get around by myself in New York, but I am at the point where I feel like everything I've packed is essential, and my bags are both still overweight. I really don't want to pay extra to check my bags, since that cost will have to come directly out of my pocket, but eventually I give up on trying to get one of them under fifty pounds. "It's just not possible," I tell Jake, exasperated. "Maybe if I tell the guy at the airport I'm a nurse, he'll check them for free."

My last night at home, Jake and I sit down to watch TV together when I remember I wanted to print my contract in case anyone at the hospital asks to see it. I go into our makeshift office to print it, and I cannot believe my eyes. At the top of my contract in dark, bold letters is the word *Brooklyn*. "BROOKLYN?" I scream when I see this. "I THOUGHT I WAS GOING TO MANHATTAN!"

"What are you yelling about?" Jake comes running into the office.

I am frantically googling the address at the top of my contract. It is, in fact, located in Brooklyn. I google the address of my Airbnb. It's located in Manhattan, just over an hour by car from the Brooklyn hospital. I specifically booked that Airbnb with the plan of walking to and from work. I'm not even old enough to rent a car, and I'm sure as hell driving halfway across the country by myself in order to have my own car with me. I hate driving.

"What am I going to do?" I wail. Tears are stinging my eyes. I shake my head in growing disbelief. How could this be? How did this happen? I search my email for all correspondence with Michelle. Finally, I find it: a screenshot of my desired contract I emailed her after our original interview. The address in that screenshot is in Manhattan. When she said, "I got you the contract you wanted," I trusted that it was, in fact, the contract I wanted. I try to think back, but I don't recall her ever saying the word "Brooklyn." We both just kept calling the hospital by its name, New York Health System, but I know from my research that there are several hospitals with the same name of New York Health System with the borough at the end of the name to provide distinction on the location. The Manhattan hospital is the only level-one trauma facility in the system. That's where I had wanted to work. My mistake or hers? Both, I decide, but it doesn't matter now.

"I'm sure you can find another Airbnb," Jake suggests. He obviously does not know what to do or how to help.

"Yeah, O.K., I guess." I start to search for one. There is seemingly nothing available within walking distance of the Brooklyn hospital. Fuck. Fuck fuck fuck fuck FUCK!

I am panicking. I go back into the living room, collapse next to Jake, and begin to cry. My sobs start out silent, but they quickly turn into blubbering. Jake is becoming visibly uneasy. He can't console me. I imagine he's trying not to have his own meltdown over the fact that, in the morning, I'll be leaving for over three months.

"Just don't go then," he offers after a while. "Just stay here. Call the recruitment lady and tell her that this isn't what you wanted, and you are not going. Problem solved!"

Problem solved? "I have to go," I tell him between sobs. "I no longer have a job. The hospital here won't take me back, and all the other ones in the area have a hiring freeze right now. Not going is no longer an option."

"I have a job. We'll be fine," he tells me, patting my shoulder and begging me with his eyes to calm down.

"O.K." I say. "Maybe I'll just email her and say I wanted the other New York Health System hospital. Maybe she can change it."

I call Michelle. She doesn't answer, so I email her instead. I try to explain what happened as best I can, and I try to be firm that I don't care how but she needs to get me a contract in Manhattan first thing in the morning.

In the email, I threaten that if she can't pull it off, I won't get on the plane, but I'm bluffing. I don't know what else to do. Sure, Jake has a job, but thanks to the pandemic, he's gone three pay periods without a paycheck. He's been stressed every other week about the uncertainty of keeping his law firm open, and before COVID-19, he was constantly stressed about the amount of credit card debt he has. So much so that I haven't told him that my credit card debt has gotten so much higher than my bi-weekly income that I can no longer afford the minimum payments. No way am I going to put all that stress on him. I've done enough in recent months, if not our entire relationship. He has credit card debt only because he helped support me while I was in nursing school and then soon after paid for our wedding.

I can't think of anything else to do, so I start on my go-to coping mechanism of the past few months: drinking. I down glasses of Woodford Reserve whiskey. First one, then two. Then I lose track, and before long I pass out drunk in our bed. I wake up sometime around 3 a.m. For some reason, my bedside lamp is on. Jake is asleep beside me, and my suitcases is open on the floor in front of us, nearly packed except for the toiletries I need to get ready with this morning. It takes me a minute to remember the woes of the previous evening.

I check my phone. No reply from Michelle. I get up and drink some water. It doesn't take long for my anxiety to reach full force again, and I lie awake re-panicking. I remember reading a devotional that said that when you can't sleep, you should try reading your Bible. *Maybe God is trying to tell you something,* it had said. Well, it can't hurt to try.

I don't want to wake Jake by digging through my suitcase for my current Bible, so I go to my bookshelf and grab the one I read from in college. I stopped using this one because it's a *New King James Version* and I found the language to be too old-timey for me to stay focused on the message. I pray as I walk back to my side of the bed: *God, I feel so lost right now. Everything is wrong. I'm starting to think You never meant for me to do this. I'm going to randomly flip this book open; please give me an answer with the page I land on.*

I close my eyes and open the Bible at random. I take a deep breath before I opened my eyes, certain that the passage I've flipped to will tell me nothing. There's a notecard between the pages, from my Dad. It says:

Believe in yourself—
In the power you have
To control your own life,

Day by day,
Believe in the strength
That you have deep inside,
And your faith will help
Show you the way.
Believe in tomorrow
And what it will bring,
Let a hopeful heart carry you through,
For things will work out if you trust and believe—
There's no limit to what you can do!

On the back is a hand-written note from him:

Laura,

Please keep this poem nearby, read it frequently, and try to understand its meaning. If you can do it, you can make your presence a positive influence wherever you go, whatever you do.

Love you so deeply,

Dad

Tears well in my eyes. *Thank you,* I whisper. *Thank you.* I go to sleep. My problems can wait until morning. I am choosing to believe in tomorrow.

WE'RE NOT IN KANSAS (CITY) ANYMORE

After a few hours sleep, I get up early and continue my search for an Airbnb in Brooklyn. I find an affordable one that has a washer and dryer and is only two miles from the hospital. I book it for two weeks. *Maybe I can find something closer once I'm out there.* Embarrassingly, I need Jake to pay for the Airbnb. We don't share our bank accounts or our personal expenses with one another, and I hate asking him for money that is for use explicitly for myself. "Thanks," I tell him. "I'll pay you back with my first paycheck."

"No worries, babe. I'm just glad you've figured something out."

Michelle calls me while I'm packing the last of my things. "Laura, hi. I got your message. I'm so sorry, but there's no way to change the contract this close to your start date. Manhattan just doesn't have any openings right now. I don't understand how this happened. The hospital address is at the top of the contract you signed."

"Yeah," I tell her, "my bad."

I signed it on my phone. So it wasn't until last night, when I printed it out, that I noticed. Since you and I have been referring to the hospital by its surname, I just assumed we were on the same page. It's O.K. now. I found a new Airbnb, and the landlord I was supposed to have in Manhattan refunded my deposit."

"O.K. good, because this is just such a wonderful opportunity for you, and such good money! I would hate to see you throw it away." Her concern for my well-being sounds genuine, but I'll later learn that agents make money off of their travel nurses, so the more money I was making, the more money Michelle was making.

Once I'm ready to go and everything is packed, we have about forty-five minutes before we need to leave. "Should we have sex?" I ask Jake, although I'm not really in the mood. The emotions of last night and this morning feel heavy. Part of me feels like we should've had something special planned for last night—a date-night in sort of thing—but I also feel like *he* should've been the one to plan it since I've been doing things to get ready to travel. Although we've only been married since September, we've been together since 2014. We aren't a very "romantic" couple anymore. The honeymoon stage ended before the proposal, I think.

"Sure," Jake says, smiling and leaning in to make out with me. It doesn't feel like he's in the mood, either, and after a while we just resolve to cuddling.

"I haven't slept by myself since we moved in together four years ago. That's going to be super weird."

"I know, babe. It's going to be weird for me, too." He seems sad, and I feel guilty for leaving. But, after finding my Dad's note last night, I also feel confident that I'm doing what I'm supposed to.

Jake drives me to the airport and helps me carry my overweight bags to the check-in. "How on Earth are you going to carry these in New York?" he asks. At sixty and eighty pounds, he can barely pull them.

"I'm not sure, but I'll have to figure it out somehow." The man at the check-in waives the oversize fee when I tell him I'm a nurse headed to New York for three months. I thank him profusely, as my personal funds are running very low. Jake walks with me to the security line. "Well," I ask him, "do you want to hang out for a little while longer, or should we just rip the Band-Aid?"

"Let's just rip the Band-Aid. I think that'll be easier."

"Yeah, me too," I agree. Jake refuses to take his mask off in the airport, even to give me a final kiss, so I hug him goodbye. I try to memorize the way his body feels pressed against mine. I thought I would cry when we parted ways, but after last night I don't have any tears left. Our goodbye feels very anticlimactic. Like this should be a big, emotional moment, but it just isn't.

We've been handling the pandemic very differently, and because of that, very separately, it feels. I still hold resentment towards him for his reaction to my first day as a COVID nurse, and I bet, if you asked him, he'd say he still holds resentment towards me, too. I feel like he hasn't been as supportive as he should be. Like this is one of those times in life where I need him to give more to our relationship because I have less to give. But he feels the same way. He's always been a bit of a germaphobe, and a pandemic is his worst nightmare. He's been wiping off our groceries with LOC, washing his hands excessively, wearing multiple masks anytime he has to go out in public, etc. I face the idea of death all the time at work, so maybe I just have a different outlook about it. I'm also religious, whereas Jake is not, so he lacks any comfort I take in the idea that a higher power is ultimately residing over my fate.

I've convinced myself that by flying to New York to work with COVID patients, I'm helping protect Jake. He won't have to worry about direct exposure from me anymore. Whether I've had this thought as a genuine concern for his safety or a vindictive "we'll-just-see-how-much-safer-life-feels-without-your-wife-around" sort of thing is unclear to me. All I know is work has been draining, and Jake and I have more or less been co-existing the past month.

I get through security in a matter of minutes. There's hardly anyone here at the airport. *What now?* I wonder. I have an hour and a half until my flight leaves. I try to read *Untamed*, but I'm too anxious to focus. I decide to browse Airbnb again since I have the time, and miraculously I find a place not even two blocks from my hospital.

I call Jake to tell him the good news. "See?" he says. "Everything is going to be O.K."

"O.K.," I tell him. I'm still not convinced, but at least my housing problem has been handled.

Brad shows up about a half hour before take-off. We laugh about having paid for priority boarding; there are maybe fifteen people on our flight. "Habit," I say, and Brad nods in agreement.

Some of the people on our plane are wearing masks; some aren't. One guy is wearing a hazmat suite. Everybody has their own row, and the first two are blocked off so that no one is sitting too close to the flight attendants. I've never been on a plane this empty.

Brad and I chat for a while, but I don't remember what we talk about. Eventually, neither of us has anything left to say. I think we're both nervous about the days ahead. At least I am. I'm nervous about the *night* ahead. I've never left an airport by myself. I'm still not sure how I'm going to get my bags from the airport to the Airbnb, or where I'll get dinner, or what the city will be like. I've been to New York once before, last winter, but that was a different world entirely. I was with Jake. He knew where to go. He knew how to handle things. Now, I feel so alone.

"I feel like there's COVID everywhere," Brad says, looking around Laguardia airport, when we get off our plane around 5 p.m.

"This is eerie," I say. "When Jake and I were here last year, this airport was so full of people we had to sit on the floor." Now, there's almost no one. The airport's shops and restaurants are all boarded up. Unlike in Kansas City, every airport employee we see is wearing a mask. We get lost more than once looking for the baggage claim. I should know where it is, I've been here before, but I'm too lost in thought and awe. We stop to take pictures of the nothingness. Finally, we find our bags.

"Do you think it'll be easier to take an Uber or a cab?" Brad asks me.

"I don't know," I say. "Jake and I took a cab, but we didn't really use Uber back then." In all honesty, I want to take an Uber. The driver of the cab Jake and I took the previous winter drove us to the wrong address after failing to understand Jake correctly. I don't want to get lost today. "Let's Uber," I decide.

The Uber wait area, it turns out, is up a long, gradual incline, quite a trek from baggage claim. I hate myself for packing as much as I have as I struggle to farmer-lunge my two suitcases behind me. A kind airport employee sees me struggling to keep up with Brad and offers me a suitcase dolly. He offers to walk us to the Uber waiting area. Brad adds his luggage to the dolly and pushes it the rest of the way. I'm relieved; it takes me the entire walk to catch my breath. I wonder how I'll possibly get my stuff from the Uber to my apartment by myself. The airport employee and Brad walk ahead of me. "Where are you from?" I hear the employee ask Brad.

"Kansas City."

"Oh wow. Long way from home. What are you doing way out here during a pandemic?"

"We're nurses," Brad answers. "We came to help."

"Oh my goodness, nurses. Thank you guys so much!" he tells us. "I can't tell you how badly we need the help. God bless you guys!"

"Thanks," Brad answers, "that's very kind of you."

We get to the Uber pick-up spot and both our cars are already there. My driver sees the size of my suitcases and offers to put them in the trunk for me. "Bless you, you beautiful man!" I tell him.

I ride in silence to my Airbnb, where my hostess has said she'll be waiting for me. I silently pray she'll offer to help with my bags. She does, and we get them up to her place with no trouble. "I wanted to help you get settled because the locks are kind of tricky if you've never seen them before," she tells me in the elevator. She lives on the eleventh floor.

I have no idea what she's talking about, I'm still so overwhelmed by my current situation, but I soon learn exactly what she means and I'm grateful she thought to explain the lock in person. It's a small, clock-looking device that lights up with tiny, touch-screen numbers. The "key" is a nine-digit code. It takes me a few tries to hit the numbers in the correct order; they're so small my fingers keep hitting the wrong ones.

She gives me a small tour of her place and tells me I'm free to help myself to anything in the fridge or cabinets. She's left some toiletries out for me in the bathroom and some chocolates on the coffee table. I thank her for everything. "You and your place are a life-saver," I tell her.

"So glad I could help!" she tells me. "Just one last thing. If any of the concierges ask, you are my friend. A guest staying with me, Taylor. Ok?"

"O.K. . . .," I say. I think this is weird, but I've never lived in a building with a concierge before.

"And whatever you do," she goes on, "don't tell them you're here through Airbnb, O.K.?" Ah, now I get it. Well, it's too late to stay anywhere else. "There's a code to get in through the side entry at the bottom of the elevators located at the end of this hall. I usually just come in that way so I don't have to talk to them."

"Yeah, O.K., sounds good," I tell her, getting the feeling she wants me to avoid talking to them, too. With that, Taylor is gone, and I am all alone in New York City.

ORIENTATION

I TAKE A BREATH. I look around the apartment, my home for the next two weeks. It's a luxury-style apartment, the kind where the kitchen is too small to even really be called one, but the living room is so big it can hold a sectional. I walk over to the window. To my right, I can see the Downtown Brooklyn skyline. I exhale as I stare at the view. It's beautiful.

I want to shower—Lord only knows what I brought in with me from the airport—but I decide it makes the most sense to get dinner first. I was planning on ordering in for dinner and trying to find a grocery store tomorrow—it's cold and nearly dark out and—but after Taylor's warning to avoid the concierge, I feel like I can't have food delivered here. I grab my mask, my license, and my debit card and venture outside.

Where I exit the apartment building, the Downtown skyline has moved to my left. To my right I see a lot of shops and a few people walking, so I decide to head that direction. I walk across the street and into a deli. The inside looks like the food section of a gas station. I go to the fridge. It's full of beer, but I see no signs of food.

The next deli I happen upon, just a few stores down, has a bigger refrigerated section. I find milk and eggs and decide that's good enough. I grab a six pack of beer as well, and on my way to the counter I grab a bag of bananas. Breakfast. Thank goodness for mandatory masks, because my mouth falls wide open when I hear the total. Forty dollars. So much for keeping the cost of food low.

I'm walking back towards my Airbnb when I pass a red doorway. It's sticking out onto the sidewalk more than the rest of the doorways are, and it looks oddly familiar. I walk a little closer. In the window I can see a menu. As I scan the menu items I begin to realize this is the same restaurant Jake and I tried on our first day in New York last January. We found it accidentally when our taxi driver got lost taking us from the airport to our hotel. He pulled over next to look up directions and I snapped a picture of the red doorway with the restaurant name on it: Belli. The sign outside advertised a truffle pasta special, and I had every intention of trying it at the earliest opportunity. Jake and I walked to it after getting settled in our hotel at about 2 p.m. We were the only ones in the restaurant. It's a memory I cherish, our first shared experience in New York City.

We thought it was a hole-in-the-wall restaurant. It definitely didn't look like a chain. Seeing it here in Brooklyn, I wonder whether it's the same one, but I realize it can't be, because Jake and I had stayed in Manhattan. I smile anyway. Chain or not, it's definitely the same restaurant, and I take it as another sign that I am exactly where I'm meant to be. I like to think God is winking at me. I feel slightly more at ease as I venture back to my Airbnb.

Once inside, I lock the door and hop straight into the shower. Feeling clean, I pop open a beer and settle onto the ledge next to the window looking out towards Downtown Brooklyn. I smile as I stare at the city lights and sip on my

Brooklyn-brewed IPA. I am fully present in this moment, and I know I am exactly where I'm supposed to be. This experience is going to change my life; I can feel it.

I wake up in a slight panic. I have no idea where I am. It's dark, and Jake isn't beside me. It takes me a minute to remember: I'm in New York. I'm alone. It's O.K. I reach for my phone. It's 3 a.m. I realize that I never did eat dinner. I must have forgotten or decided I didn't care enough to bother after drinking my beer. I remember I didn't drink any water either. I called Jake to ask whether it was safe to drink the tap water after an inconclusive Google search. He didn't think it was, either. I had forgotten to pick some up from the deli,—I never buy bottled water at home (save the polar bears!)—and I didn't want to go out again after showering. I planned to get some first thing the next morning, but now it's 3 a.m. and I'm parched.

Taylor told me to help myself to any of the "eats," and she just so happens to have a bottle of San Pellegrino in the fridge. Good enough. I look at the skyline as I drink it: still shining. I look around the apartment: still alone. It's unnerving. I watch a couple episodes of *The Office* before I'm able to fall back asleep.

Later that week, on Wednesday, we have online orientation. The hospital is bringing on about 100 travel nurses at once, and it isn't safe to have that many people in one room. The orientation is standard stuff, like what color scrubs to wear (any, because that's the least of the hospital's worries right now), where to park, where to go to on our in-person orientation day, etc. We've been split into smaller groups for our in-person orientation. Mine is on Friday.

During the online orientation, someone mentions that Citi Bike is giving a free month pass to nurses, so I sign up for one. I spend Thursday biking to and from the hospital a few times to make sure I know where I'm going and how long it takes. I don't want to be late for my first day just because I got lost, and I have a pretty long track record for getting lost. I'm fortunate enough to have a bike dock right outside my Airbnb, and there's another one directly in front of the hospital. It's about a two mile trip one-way, with a bike lane available for the whole trip.

Before I know it, it's Friday. I wake up early to make eggs and toast for breakfast. Getting ready takes me no time at all. My hair is braided back into a scrub cap, and I've stopped wearing any makeup other than mascara. With a mask on, you can't see anything other than my eyes. I leave about twenty minutes earlier than I need to—just to be sure I'm on time. The bike ride takes me less time than it did yesterday; no one is out this early. I am still not used to the quiet hours of New York; I don't think they existed pre-COVID. I listen to some up-beat music to try to get pumped for the day ahead as the crisp morning air helps to wake me and clear my head. I'm nervous; I don't know what to expect for today. I wish I packed gloves.

The first half of the day is a continuation of a general hospital orientation. About forty or fifty of us are brought into an auditorium and told to sit a few seats apart from each other. I settle into a seat on the edge.

"Welcome to New York Health System of Brooklyn," the presenter says. I can't remember her official title, just that she's someone important. "Thank you all so much for being here.

I'm proud to announce that you are the third wave of travel nurses we've brought on board. We have desperately needed your help, and once you all start working, I believe our hospital will *finally* be able to say it has adequate staffing for the situation at hand. You guys chose the right contract. I'm also proud to say that we have more than enough PPE. Each day you will be given a fresh N95 mask, and there is no limit to the number of gowns you can use. The only thing that we ask you reuse is the face shields we're passing out now. Put your name on it, and don't lose it."

After hearing that they have more protective gear than my previous hospital, I completely agree that I chose the right contract. I take the presenter's statement as another wink from God. She goes on to ask us to please be understanding and kind to the hospital's staff nurses. "In the past few weeks, months even, they have had to deal with short staffing and an overwhelming amount of patients and patient deaths. Some of them have been sick. Some of them have family members who have been sick. They are exhausted, and while we all greatly appreciate you guys coming here to help, it's also added work for them to show you how to do things and where to find supplies. So please, be as compassionate to our nurses as we know you all are to your patients."

I bet they all know we're getting paid a lot more than they are, too, I think. I doubt I'd like having to deal with a bunch of travel nurses asking me questions. I'm just thankful to be the annoying travel nurse and not the overworked staff nurse anymore.

We spend the next hour reviewing the hospital's charting system. If I got a dollar for every time the man presenting says "But, due to the COVID situation," I would make some overtime. He explains the hospital policies regarding charting, and then reexplains the charting requirements for the "COVID situation." Thanks to special orders from Governor Cuomo, we don't have to chart with the usual detail required by legal and hospital policies. There just isn't time. I've always said that my patients would receive much better care if I didn't have to waste so much time charting every little thing I do. Besides, nurses don't want to chart things or type on a computer. We want to help people. I'm excited to hear I will get to see my theory in practice.

Our group is divided into three smaller groups. Each is taken to a room to learn how to use the hospital equipment and make sure we can log on to the computer system. Then it's time to go to work. Each travel nurse is dropped off onto a different floor. There are three actual ICUs and three make-shift ICUs. The make-shift ICU's have taken over the psychiatric floor, the cath lab, and the pediatric ICU. I get to orient on one of the original ICUs.

The manager of the unit reexplains the loose charting requirements on his way to drop me off. "Just chart what you can, and make sure each patient has an assessment and a set of vital signs charted. Charting is the least of our worries right now; just try not to let patients die." After a short pause he adds, "And if they do, oh well. We're all doing the best we can right now." Wow. What am I in for?

Surprisingly, it's a pretty chill day. The unit is adequately staffed this shift, and the nurse I'm assigned to has herself only been assigned to one patient. She spends most of the afternoon trying to show me where things are on the unit, so I won't have to ask where they are when I'm on my own. She's nice but appears uninterested in chatting. I'm O.K. with this; I'm just taking it all in.

*****

They tell me my first official day will be Monday, so I have the weekend off. I make plans to meet up with Maddi and walk around the city a bit. We decide to cross the Brooklyn Bridge to see the 9/11 Memorial. When we get there, we are sad to learn that the fountains are roped off and not running "due to COVID-19." I've seen them before. Last January, when Jake and I visited, we went to the 9/11 Museum. We looked at the fountains, too, but it was minus-four degrees outside, so we didn't look for very long.

Jake has recently told me about an article he read stating that New York has officially lost more people to COVID-19 than they did to 9/11. I share this with Maddi. We stand in silence for a while. I look down at the depth of the memorial fountains. My mind sees stacks of dead bodies filling the fountain, reaching up towards the top of One World Trade Center to my right. I was only six years old when 9/11 happened, so I barely remember it, but I know already that that image of bodies is burned in my mind for life.

THROWN IN THE DEEP END

BEFORE I KNOW IT, IT'S Monday. *Time to kick some COVID ass.* I play pump-up music during my bike ride to work again. I have no idea what to expect. I get assigned to one of the make-shift ICUs. The doors are wooden, and there are two patients per room. Both things are normally unheard of in the ICU. I'm used to glass doors with big monitors so I can see my patients at all times and respond immediately to any vital-sign changes. Here, I will have to rely on the monitor nurse to tell me when my patient's vitals warrant my attention. I am assigned a psychiatric nurse, Jeff, to help me. "I can give medications, chart vital signs, and help with turns. All the IV medications and other ICU-level stuff is on you," Jeff says. Having an extra set of hands that is readily available is a new concept to me. One I will soon realize I could not survive my day without.

Both my patients are here because they have COVID-19. I am told that every patient on this floor has tested positive. They are both in their sixties, intubated, and on multiple pressers. I'm only thirty minutes into my shift when a doctor informs me that one of my patients, the one in bed A, is going to need CVVHD today. At my previous hospital, those patients were strictly one-on-one with their nurse, but here that's not even an option. I'm glad I learned how to do CVVHD before I came out here. Hopefully, I'll be able to trouble-shoot any alarms the machine has today.

Usually, when I'm assigned two patients, one is notably sicker than the other. When the doctor tells me the patient in bed A is going to require CVVHD, I assume that makes her the sickest. I have barely had enough time to consider this when the patient in bed B has a significant drop in blood pressure. I titrate up slightly on one of her blood pressure medications, and no sooner do I think I've fixed the problem than her systolic blood pressure shoots from tanking in the sixties up to the two-hundreds. *What the fuck? I only went up by two micrograms. That's a textbook titration!* I pause the medication and beg her blood pressure to come back down. After a few minutes, it drops back to a normal pressure. I turn to leave the room when the monitor nurse says over the radio, "Laura, bed B is hypotensive again." I turn around, and sure enough the patient's blood pressure critically low, right back where it started.

I titrate the medication up by one microgram. I watch her blood pressure start to soar to the 200s. I pause the pressor. I watch her blood pressure plummet to potential death. I truly, truly wish I was exaggerating when I say that I spend the next *four* hours of my day like this, but I'm not. I've never seen anything quite like it before. Patients are never this sensitive to pressers when they are this reliant on them to survive. A couple hours into this routine of chasing my patient's blood pressure, I radio the monitor nurse to explain the situation and ask whether there's anything else she thinks I should do. No one here has worked with me before, and I'm afraid they've all been watching the monitor wondering whether I have the first clue what I'm doing.

"Nope, you're doing good," she says. "They told me she did that for a while last night. Hopefully she'll cut it out soon. Do you need anything? Is your other patient O.K.?"

As if she heard the monitor nurse and realized she wasn't causing problems, the patient in bed A has a drop in blood pressure. *You've got to be kidding me.* I titrate her presser up by one microgram and am met with the same problem. *Thank God they're in the same room.* I pull back the curtain that's separating them; I need to be able to see both monitors at once. I pull both IV poles to the center of the room so I can reach them simultaneously. It doesn't take long for me to feel like I'm playing Whac-A-Mole as my patients' blood pressures yo-yo simultaneously for the next two hours.

Finally, they both remain stable for more than ten minutes and I get a chance to leave the room. I'm met at the door by the monitor nurse. "Oh my gosh, are you O.K.?" she asks. "You've been in there for four straight hours. You should get some water and some food. I'll watch your patients for you. I promise I won't let either of them tank."

Four hours? That can't be right. I look at the clock. 12:10 p.m. *Holy crap.* "Yeah, O.K. Thank you," I say

After a power bar and a couple bottles of water, I'm feeling much better. The calm doesn't last long, though; it seldom does. The physicians inform me they're going to place a line for temporary dialysis on the patient in bed A now that she's better stabilized. *Of course we are.* "Do we really think that's going to help?" I ask. "She's on three pressors. At my last hospital, that fact alone deemed a patient too unstable for CVVHD. More likely than not, as soon as I start dialysis her blood pressure is going to re-tank."

"We're aware," one of the physicians says "But we've contacted the family several times today to explain the situation, and they still want everything done. Without the dialysis, her potassium level is going to kill her."

And with the dialysis, her blood pressure, or lack thereof, is going to kill her. I sigh. It's not up to me.

Once they finish placing the dialysis line, the physicians order a new set of labs to make sure the patient's blood volume is high enough for her to tolerate the dialysis. The lab calls back shortly after I've sent them to inform us that the patient's hemoglobin value is three.

Three? How is that even possible? A normal hemoglobin level is twelve to seventeen, and blood replacement is typically ordered for a hemoglobin of less than seven. The physicians and I are all confused. We check the patient, but there are no obvious signs of bleeding. Her hemoglobin was 7.6 with her morning labs. That's a lot of blood to lose in seven hours with no visible signs of bleeding, although it would help explain why she's needed such a large increase in blood pressure support this shift. Normally, we would do a C.T. scan in attempt to locate an internal bleed, but this patient is way too unstable to move, thus deeming a C.T. unsafe.

"We're going to have to start massive transfusion protocol immediately," the PA tells me.

Great. I have no idea how that works here.

"O.K.," Kelly, the charge nurse, says. "I'll call ICU and get the rapid infuser. Jeff, you go to blood bank and get the cooler. Laura, you get as much gravity tubing as you can find and push fluids until we get back to help replace your patient's blood volume." I say a silent thank-you for all the help, and for the fact that someone more knowledgeable about the hospital's policies and procedures is taking charge of the situation for me.

Within twenty minutes, everyone is outside my patient's room with the supplies. The ICU manager even came up with Kelly in case we need the extra hands. "Plus, I really like using the rapid infuser," she tells me with a wink. I'm relieved to see that it's the same rapid infuser we used in Kansas City. I had a patient who required it while I worked there, so I've used it before. Sometimes in the ICU, half the battle is knowing how to use the machinery. Kelly and I get to work. The name rapid infuser is very accurate; in the few minutes it takes Kelly to scan a bag of blood, the bag that's hanging has already been pushed into the patient. I'm now thankful the physicians decided to place a dialysis catheter. They are much bigger than central lines, providing me with the perfect line for a blood transfusion, especially one running this fast.

We've frantically pushed all but one blood product in the MTP cooler when the PA tells us that the family has finally decided to make the patient a DNR. Almost the minute the final blood product is transfused, the patient's blood pressure starts to tank. Kelly and I were continuously titrating up on the patient's BP medications while we were transfusing, and they are now maxed out. There is quite literally nothing we can do about the falling blood pressure. I watch the screen in disbelief as the patient's blood pressure and then heart rate sink down to zero within minutes. We've done so much work to try to keep her alive. It's past 4 p.m. I've been trying to save her since I got here at 7:30, and now she's just *gone*.

"Well," Kelly tells me as she, too, stands there helplessly, "you know how we tell families 'We did everything we could'? You have literally done everything and then some for this patient today. There was nothing more to do. You did a good job. Get some lunch. We can do postmortem care when you get back."

I know Kelly is right, but I'm still shocked. The fact that she died the very minute the last of the blood products went into her system, and the minute after her family made her a DNR, feels like a cruel joke. In hindsight, I now wonder whether the patient heard the physician say that her family had made her a DNR and took that as a sign that she was allowed to let go. When you see death as often as I have, you learn that patients who are near death often hang on or let go for a reason. I've seen patients wait for the last family member to make it to the hospital, wait for their loved ones to verbally give them permission to go, or die while their family was on the way to the hospital as if to spare them the sight of their death.

I'm moving much more slowly after lunch. I feel both defeated and depleted. 4:30 p.m. was the first time I sat down all day, and I didn't realized how tired I was until I stopped moving. Not to mention that it's depressing to lose a fight against death. The PA was also in disbelief when we told her the patient expired. "Her family is going to think we stopped trying the minute they made her a DNR," she said. There is often a misconception that DNR means "do not treat." This could not be further from the truth. DNR stands for Do Not Resuscitate, meaning we will do everything we possibly can to prevent a heart from stopping, but if it *does* stop, we will not do compressions in an attempt to restart it. We will often advocate for patients who we know will not survive compressions, like my patient today, to become DNRs so that we do not have to put their dying body through the trauma of a code. CPR is violent. It breaks the ribs, and the person performing chest compressions is manually pumping that person's heart for them. For patients like mine today, we know that if multiple blood pressure medications and a ventilator can't keep the heart beating, pumping it manually isn't going to restart it. There truly is only so much we can do.

I'm worried that the minute I complete postmortem care, I'm going to be given an admission. That was how the COVID unit seemed to operate at my last hospital. I'm both physically and emotionally exhausted, and I pray that another patient will not come. My prayers are answered. Security doesn't even come to take the body to the morgue until the end of my shift. I barely have time to do basic care on the patient in bed B by the time we get the room and the patient in bed A cleaned up. I feel lousy. The patient in bed B looks like she could use a bath, but I don't have the time. I hope whoever's on night shift does.

I get on the elevator to leave the same time as the PA. She looks defeated. "Are you back tomorrow?" she asks me.

"Yeah, are you?"

"Yeah. Let's hope tomorrow isn't this crazy."

"Amen to that," I say. "Sorry that family gave you such a hard time."

"It's O.K.," she says. "They don't understand everything we tried to explain to them, and it's hard to feel confident that medical professionals really are doing everything when you don't know what 'everything' entails and you can't be present to see everything being done. It's nice that visitors aren't physically in our way right now, but it's hard, too, because they aren't able to see everything that's going on. Sometimes seeing all the machines and people in the room helps them understand what they aren't able to comprehend just from explanation. And I think families are fighting harder than before to keep their loved ones alive because they're so torn up about the fact that they can't say goodbye. I can't blame them. I can't imagine having a loved one die alone."

I think of my Dad. I'm grateful this was not his fate. I pray that my patient's family can find peace. I also pray that the PA beside me can forgive herself for their grief. I pray I can forgive myself, too. If every shift is like this one, I'm in for a very long thirteen weeks.

BAGELS AND BATH TIME

THE NEXT DAY PROVES TO be a little kinder. It begins with free bagels and coffee brought to the hospital by one of the psychiatric nurses for the travel nurses assigned to his floor today to thank us for coming to New York to help fight COVID. Despite the fact that his psychiatric unit is now overrun with ICU COVID-positive patients, despite the fact that he now has to work as a glorified nurse tech for travel nurses on his own unit, despite the fact that he knows we are making four times as much money per hour as he is to be here to work, he has taken some of the money he has earned to buy us breakfast so we feel welcome and appreciated. I hope he knows how much this gesture means to me. I can't help but think that if I were him, I'd be too pissed off to come to work, let alone to buy the foreigners bagels.

Jeff is my helper nurse again and we are assigned only one patient today, the one from bed B the previous day. Bed A is still unoccupied. *Thank God, I can give her that bath she desperately needs.*

Once we've started, it feels impossible to stop. When we bathe the patient, I realize her many dressings need to be changed. I decide we might as well change her bed linens, too. When we turn her to change the fitted sheet, I notice that the hair on the back of her head is extremely matted. I tell Jeff we should try to wash and comb it.

This proves to be easier said than done. Her hair is so matted that sometimes when we tug hard enough on the knots to break them up, we also pull small chunks of hair off her head. The monitor nurse, Ulga, is the same one as yesterday, and she keeps popping in to ask whether we need help or want to take a break. I tell her we're O.K.

"You've been in there for nearly four hours, just like yesterday," she says tentatively.

"I know," I reply, "but I really want to get this done, and if I end up getting another patient, that won't happen. She needed this done weeks ago."

As Jeff and I move from the sides of the patient's hair to the middle, I see blood. I realize it's not being caused by our combing. It's old, dried blood from what appears to be, upon further inspection, a rather large wound. "Are you fucking kidding me?" I say to Jeff. "Has she really been laying in this position for so long that there's now a pressure wound on her *head*?"

"That would appear to be the case, yes. Shit, that's messed up."

"I mean, I know everyone's been busy and overworked and overwhelmed, and I realize she's not exactly doing superb, but, like, this is ridiculous. These are people. These are fucking human beings and they have enough shit to deal with without us giving them head wounds. I bet you anything the doctors are going to tell us to shave her head around this wound so it can heal. And it's huge. If or when she wakes up, how do you think that's going to make her feel? Jesus Christ."

I'm don't usually take the Lord's name in vain, but I'm feeling particularly exasperated, and I'm still a bit emotionally exhausted and overwhelmed from yesterday. Sure enough, once the PA sees the wound, he says we will have to shave the surrounding area, apply antibiotic ointment, and do our best to keep the patient's head elevated on a donut pillow to alleviate further pressure. It's nearly 1 p.m.

"I'll cut her hair and find a donut pillow. Why don't you take a lunch break before it turns into a dinner break like yesterday," Jeff offers.

"Yeah, O.K. That's probably a good idea. Thanks." I think he can tell I'm losing my marbles a bit faster than I did yesterday. If I even have any left to lose.

Sure enough, when I come back from lunch we get an admission. Ulga tells me the patient is being admitted for a stroke.

"Then why are we getting her?" I ask. "Our other patient is intubated and COVID positive. A COVID-negative patient can't share a room with her."

"Well, I'm pretty sure she's COVID positive, too, but she's also had a stroke."

And both of those things happened at the same time? It just doesn't make sense to me. Either she's recently had a stroke *and* she's being admitted for COVID, or she's recently had COVID and she's being admitted for a stroke. I try to log on to a computer to read the doctor's ED note to get a better idea of why this patient is being admitted, but for some reason Ulga feels the need to be involved. She keeps pushing my hands out of the way to search through the chart herself, and she keeps repeating that she's been told this patient is being admitted for

COVID and a stroke. I'm perturbed, and I keep exchanging glances with Jeff that say as much.

Finally, I get to the bottom of things. The patient, Martha, has recently suffered a stroke, and she's now being admitted for worsening COVID symptoms. *That* makes sense to me. That diagnosis I know how to care for. Martha comes to us around 5 p.m. She's on ten liters of oxygen, and the ED nurse tells me that she hasn't been very responsive or communicative. She's coming to the ICU because she is going to need CVVHD. Once I get her settled and assessed, the residents get to work placing a temporary dialysis catheter. Luckily, its late enough in my shift that I won't have to start dialysis. That responsibility will fall to night shift.

After they're done, I go in to see how Martha's doing and finish my end-of-shift tasks for her roommate. She tells me she's very upset that she has to share a room. I sympathize with her, but I tell her there is nothing I can do, hers is the only ICU bed we had available. I can't imagine how scary it must be to look over and see someone half-dead from a disease that you now have. To see someone lying there, lifeless, with a tube jammed down their throat to help them breathe and a donut pillow under their head, exposing a gnarly wound. To be confused, due to a recent stroke, about everything that is going on, and to not be able to have a family member visit or help explain things. To look up at all the people claiming they are here to help you from behind multiple masks, glasses, gowns, and gloves. To be told that you're in intensive care because the virus you've contracted is killing your kidneys. To be unable to breathe without a mask blowing oxygen on your face. To be hungry but unable to eat because your body can't tolerate taking the oxygen mask off long enough for a decent meal. I truly can't imagine, and try as I might, I am unable to make the situation much better for her. None of the scary things on that list can be eradicated or changed.

I've only been here two days, and already my heart is heavy with the phrase I utter to Martha: "I'm sorry, but I can't fix that."

THE MOVE TO PARK SLOPE

THAT SATURDAY IS MY ONE day off between my first and second week of work, and it's moving day for me. A few days into my stay at this downtown apartment, I found a different Airbnb that's only one block away from my hospital. Although I've kind of grown to enjoy my daily bike rides to and from the hospital, I'm excited to move within walking distance. There's a pharmacy across the street from the hospital, and a grocery store a few blocks down the road. There's also a park called Park Slope a few blocks up from where I'll be staying, so maybe I can start running again on my days off. I've considered it a few times since I've arrived, but I wasn't sure it would be safe to run through downtown Brooklyn.

I struggle once again with my two giant suitcases. The Uber driver helps me load and unload them, but once we arrive at my new Airbnb, I'm on my own. My new apartment is up two flights of stairs. The building is an old brownstone, so there's no elevator. *Here goes nothing.* I essentially have to deadlift each suitcase up one stair at a time. When I'm through, I'm huffing and sweating, but I feel accomplished. *I can totally do things by myself.*

My new apartment is perfect. As nice as the downtown Airbnb was, this one feels much homier. It's a studio unit, with a bookshelf separating the bed from the big chair that is the "living room." The kitchen is almost as big as the main room, and then there's a tiny "hallway" back to the bathroom. There's a desk against the wall at the end of the bed, which I decide will function perfectly as a vanity. The TV is huge, probably sixty inches, and easily turns, so I'll be able to watch it from either the chair or the queen-size bed. I like that there's a bookshelf in between. I put the ten books I've brought with me on the bookshelf. I place the framed pictures of me and my dad, and me and Jake, on top of it, so I can see them no matter where I am in the apartment. And just like that, it feels a little more like home.

The next morning, I walk into work accompanied by the sound of the neighborhood cheering and banging pots and pans out their windows or from their front stoop. The experience is surreal. It makes me feel like the whole town is fighting this disease, not just me. There's a little boy, who can't be older than three or four, across the street from my building standing on the front stoop and yelling at the top of his lungs a very drawn out, "Thank yooooooou!" I decide that today, I'm working for him.

WHAT (AND I CANNOT STRESS THIS ENOUGH) THE FUCK?

I'M ASSIGNED TO THREE INTUBATED patients. I'm sure this will be manageable with a helper-nurse like Jeff, but I am quickly disappointed to learn that the nurse assigned to me, Trisha, has never been on this floor and isn't happy about being here.

"If you could please just make sure to give these two patients their medications and record their vital signs," I tell her, "I'll take care of the other one and any IV drips. Gloria's really sick, so I imagine I'll be stuck in her room most often." I'm not wrong. As if to add an exclamation point to my sentence, the monitor nurse radios that Gloria's blood pressure is dropping.

I run into her room to titrate up her blood pressure meds. I stand by for a moment, expecting her blood pressure to yo-yo like it did with my two patient's the other day; it does. I pause the blood pressure meds long enough to get her systolic number—the top number of the blood pressure, which measures the force one's heart is exerting on the walls of the arteries with each beat, and most often the one health care providers try to maintain when patients require blood pressure support medications—down from the 200s to about 150 and then restart them. It stabilizes around seventy, so I titrate up a little bit more. I want that top number to stabilize somewhere around ninety to 100. It takes me hours of this back-and-forth titrating to accomplish such a number.

During these few hours, a nurse named Lucy keeps radioing me about Gregory, my patient next door. Her patient is sharing a room with Gregory, so she's been in there a lot. I have yet to see him since I got report from the night shift nurse. I also haven't seen my other patient, Richard, since report this morning. I really hope Trisha is meeting his needs. I haven't seen her since report this morning, either. "He's really awake," Lucy tells me via radio. "I'm starting to worry that he's going to manage to self-extubate. You really need to get some sedation for him."

"Um . . .O.K.," I radio back. "Thanks. I'm kind of stuck in the room next door. I can't seem to get her blood pressure to stabilize. But I'll try to get the residents to come take a look at Gregory."

I titrate up Gloria's blood pressure meds, knowing I will have to deal with the yo-yo-ing once more when I return. After ripping off my isolation gown, I speed-walk back to the residents' room. "Hey, who has Gregory?" I ask them.

"I do," says a male resident.

"Great, I don't have a ton of time, my other patient isn't doing well, but one of the other nurses told me he needs sedation. I guess he's pretty awake and she's afraid he might pull out his tube."

"Well, what do you think?" he asks me.

"I honestly haven't been in his room since report. I literally haven't left my other patients' room until now. She's really not doing well. I need help. Can you please just take a look at Gregory? Lucy, the nurse I mentioned, has the other patient in

Gregory's room. She's in there. Just ask her if you have any questions, and either radio me or pop into the room next door if you want to talk to me. Thanks." I leave before he can object.

As I race back to my patient's room, I pass another nurse who introduces herself as Emma. "Let me know if you need anything, O.K.?" she offers.

"O.K. I will. Thanks," I say as I keep running back to Gloria's room. I throw on a new isolation gown and a fresh pair of gloves and walk in to find that not only are her blood pressure numbers dropping again, but her oxygen saturation is dropping, too. In addition to her heart's inability to provide blood perfusion throughout her body, her lungs are now giving out. I pick up my radio. "Emma, I need you."

Within seconds, she's at the door of my room. "What can I do?" she asks.

"Get me the respiratory therapist and bring the crash cart in here. I think I'm about to need it."

"I'm on it."

Emma disappears, and I wrack my brain for what to do. It's anyone's guess as to whether my patient's lungs or heart will give out first, but one will definitely cause the other, and both will result in a code. On a whim, I pause her paralytic and her sedative. Even though her blood pressure is low, we have to have her on these medications in order to properly ventilate her. She's requiring so much ventilation that without the paralytic, her body would reject the forces of air it's getting from the ventilator. I know, however, that these medications cause decreased blood pressure, and I think that maybe if I pause them for a few minutes, I can get her blood pressure to recover, and that just *might* fix her ventilation, too. It's a hail Mary.

Not a lot happens when I pause those medications, but that's a good thing/bad thing. Good that she doesn't have ventilator dyssynchrony (meaning her body is still allowing the ventilator to breathe for her). Bad because there is no immediate effect on her blood pressure. I leave the sedatives and paralytics paused. Emma comes in with the crash cart, and I grab a vial of epi. I get it ready to push it. The residents trail in behind her. I give them a brief update. I tell them I'm on top of the medications but they need to do something to the vent. I have limited knowledge of how the settings affect oxygenation, and I've exhausted everything I know to do. Emma helps me roll my patient onto a backboard in case we need to do compressions, and the motion causes Gloria's heart rate to plummet. *Shit.* I grab the vial of epi and slam it into her IV. Her heart rate overreacts, shooting up well into the hundreds. Better than a zero. I titrate past the max on her blood pressure medications to push that up, too. It works. I know they're both going to drop down once the initial rush of medication passes, but it buys us a minute, and that's all we really need.

I prep another epi vial just in case. The residents are working with the respiratory therapist to try to find a ventilator setting that will get her oxygen saturation back up to an acceptable level. Every minute that her saturation is less than 92% she risks brain damage.

I'm listening to the residents' conversation and watching for her vitals to start dropping again when Lucy comes over the radio. "Hey, I know you have a lot going on next door so I'm going to go ahead and start this Precedex they ordered for Gregory."

"Oh shoot, I should've mentioned to the resident no Precedex. Gregory had a couple bouts of bradycardia last night. That's why they didn't start any sedation. They had to give atropine twice."

"Oh, O.K., good to know. I'll ask the resident if we can give something else."

"Thank you! I'm so sorry. I just can't leave this room."

"I know, it's O.K. I'll handle it."

"Thank you so, so much. Keep me updated. I'll get over there as soon as I can."

"Hey, you're doing a great job," Emma tells me.

"Thanks, I'm trying."

My patient's heart rate plummets again after the respiratory therapist makes some sort of change in the ventilator settings. I slam in half a vial of epi. I don't want to yo-yo her heart rate too much; pushing epi too many times could make it more difficult for her to recover. I end up pushing the other half after the respiratory therapist makes a different ventilator change, but this change seems to finally stabilize her oxygenation.

"O.K.," the respiratory therapist says to me and the residents, "I have her on a three-to-one setting. I'll be honest, I've never really had to put anyone on this high of a ratio before, but it seems to be the only thing she's responding to."

I have no idea what a three-to-one ratio is. I ask, but I don't understand her answer. However, the residents seem pleased, and Gloria's heart rate and blood pressure seem to be less labile now that her oxygen saturation is coming up, so I'm happy.

After another half hour of vigilant bedside monitoring and IV titrations, she seems stable. I go next door to *finally* see my other patient. It's 11:30 a.m. Lucy isn't in the room, but I can see that Versed, a sedative, is running at a low rate, and Gregory seems to be resting comfortably. I do an assessment, and as I'm done listening to his lungs, I see his heart rate start to drop. I stop what I'm doing, but I don't panic. The night-shift nurse told me this happened a few times and said I should only get excited if his heart rate dropped below thirty beats per minute. As I stare at the monitor, Gregory's heart rate goes from thirty to flatline in a matter of moments. I can't believe it.

I don't normally do the part of CPR where you shake the patient and try to rouse them, but in my exhaustion and exasperation, basic training overrides thinking. I feel for a pulse: nothing. I shake his shoulders lightly, and then violently, as I will him not to code. "Gregory?"

A short pause; no reaction.

Slightly louder this time: "Gregory?"

Still nothing.

"GREGORY, WHAT THE FUCK?" I scream as I violently shake his upper body. I reach over for the vial of atropine the night nurse left on his bedside table, determined not to do compressions, when suddenly his heart rate shoots from zero to the 160s and slowly stabilizes back down to the eighties. I hold my breath as I hold the atropine vial, frozen in place. I beg his heart to hold a rate in the eighties, and it does. I exhale loudly. "Don't do that again," I say in a stern voice as I turn to leave the room. "I need to go back next door and make sure her vitals are still O.K."

When I come out of Gregory's room, several nurses are staring at me through the glass windows of the telemetry-monitor room.

"Are you O.K.?" Emma asks me.

"Yeah," I answer nonchalantly. "He tried to die, but I screamed at him and somehow it worked."

"I'm sorry, you did what?" Kelly asks, laughing.

"Didn't you see her on the monitor camera?" Emma asks Kelly. "What did you say?"

I reenact the situation for everyone in the monitor room. By the time I say "GREGORY WHAT THE FUCK?" everyone is crying from laughing so hard.

"He probably saw the light and then heard you screaming and started as if waking from a bad dream," Kelly says between bouts of hysteria. "That's hilarious!"

"Well, hell," chimes in Emma, "if nothing else works, I guess just curse at them."

I pop back into Gloria's room to find that her vitals are still holding steady. I tell the monitor nurse that I'm going to go assess my third patient, Richard, who's inconveniently located at the other end of the hall, and to please radio me if anything starts to trend down on Gloria's vitals. I find Trisha in Richard's room. "Hey, how's he doing?" I ask her.

"He's fine. He doesn't respond to much, but I made sure he got all of his morning meds."

"Thank you so much. I'm sorry I haven't really been around, but our patient at the other end of the hall has been toying with death all morning."

"No problem." She leaves and I do my assessment. Richard is essentially a potato. He doesn't respond neurologically, and he requires a ventilator to breathe and tube feeds to eat. He has stage-four cancer and COVID-19. Even if he were to survive the COVID, his cancer can't be far from killing him. The night-shift nurse told me that these things have been explained to his wife, but she refuses to let him go. She's delusional under the notion that we might let him go home to pass away—but he's far too sick to transport—and she refuses to let him get comfort care in the hospital. It's sad, but there's nothing we can do. So, on he exists.

When I emerge from Richard's room, there's a small cluster of people outside of Gloria's room. "Hey," I say to Emma as I reach her end of the hall, "what's going on? Who are all these people?"

"Apparently, your patient's daughter works here on the seventh floor. She visits every day when the attending comes by to get an update."

"Oh, Christ. Of course, I get the one patient that gets visitors. And *of course* she's my sickest."

"I know. I'm sorry. I'm here if you need me."

"Thanks, Emma. I don't know how I would be surviving today without you."

Visitors still aren't allowed in the hospital, so I'm slightly appalled that we're making an exception for Gloria's daughter just because she works here. It seems unfair to all the other daughters stuck on the outside, willing to give anything for one more moment with their mom. I can't judge too harshly, though. If this were my Dad, I would absolutely be breaking the no-visitors rule if there was a way, and I wouldn't be thinking about those other daughters.

I enter the room. The daughter has noticeable tears welling in her eyes. Her mom is in bad shape. We haven't taken the back board out from under her, because turning her to put it there really dropped her blood pressure. The crash cart is still in the room, just in case I end up needing it again. She looks like she badly needs a bath and a bed change. I hadn't really noticed before now. The doctor is explaining that she almost coded this morning but she's stable for now. He gently suggests to the daughter that Gloria's time is near, and that she may want to reconsider further efforts at treatment, but he and

I can both tell that the daughter is in no state to hear this. He leaves the room.

"I don't understand how this happened," the daughter tells me. "Yesterday she was doing slightly better, and they were telling me she was well enough to be entered into a COVID-19 drug trial. Today she's almost dying and too sick to be a participant? What happened?"

"I'm not sure. I've only been with her since 7:30 this morning, and she's been this sick since I got here. This can just happen, though. The body can only sustain itself on these medications for so long before it starts to give out. Without these IV medications, her heart would stop pumping. And without this ventilator, her lungs would stop breathing. I don't want to upset you, but I don't want to give you false hope, either. She's not in good shape. We're doing everything we can, but her oxygen saturation dropped to the sixties for almost an hour this morning. There's a chance that even if she did recover from COVID, that hour of decreased oxygenation led to permanent brain damage. Every time that happens, her quality of life after this is going to decrease."

If I've learned anything from two years of ICU nursing, it's that doctors always tiptoe around the subjects of death and probable poor outcomes. I understand why; they don't want families to think that they're condemning their loved one, or that they're not trying to save them because they believe they are a lost cause. Thoughts like that could lead families to blame a physician for the unavoidable death of their loved ones. I would never want to cause a family to distrust their physician, but it sucks to be the one to have to come in and tell it how it is. I've lost track of the number of times I've said something along the lines of what I'm saying now. "I don't want to upset you," I say again, "but I don't want to sugar coat the situation.

Gloria's chances are slim, and it's possible that all the things we're doing to keep her alive are causing her great pain. You may want to consider ceasing treatment."

The daughter is crying now. "Please, God, not today. Not today. Not today . . ."

Those words tell me my efforts aren't going to accomplish anything, and I switch from realist to psychologist. "O.K., it's O.K. It's O.K." I know fully well it is *not* O.K. "She's stable for now, O.K.? And I'm going to do everything I possibly can to keep her that way."

"I understand what you're saying, and I *want* to stop. God, I want *all of this* to be over. But I can't do it. I can't be the one who kills my mom. My siblings don't understand. They don't work in healthcare, and they're convinced that, with enough prayers, we can have a miracle. I'm the youngest. The only reason I'm the durable power of attorney is because I'm the one who works in healthcare. I can't lose my mom and my siblings, and if I let go of my mom, my siblings would never forgive me. And yesterday the doctors were telling me that she might qualify for a drug trial, and today they're saying she's too sick. I don't understand how this keeps happening. She keeps getting worse."

"I understand, and I can't begin to imagine the pressure you must be under right now."

"I just want this nightmare to be over," she nearly whispers.

"I'm going to tell you something, and I want you to know that I'm telling you this not to get sympathy, but to let you know that I truly do understand how difficult all this is, and I care just as much as you do. I lost my Dad last August. I'm his youngest kid, and I was the DPoA, too. He was in the ICU on the same blood pressure medications your mom is on now.

This is incredibly difficult to deal with. But I want you to have confidence that, to me, your mom is my Dad. And I'm going to care for her like I would have cared for him, O.K.? I want you to know how important your mom is to us, and that we're not going to provide her with anything other than the best care. So that's one less thing you have to worry about."

She burst into tears and hugged me. "Thank you," she tells me over and over again. In this moment, it's all she can manage to say.

I hold her—gowns, gloves, and masks between us—and let her cry for a couple minutes. When she gathers her wits, she says she hopes it's not too much trouble, but could I please change her mother's gown at some point today. "I know it's the least of your worries, but every time I come in here she seems messy and unkempt. I visited last night before I went to my shift, and the night nurse didn't seem to know much about how she was doing. Her gown has had this stain on it since 10 o'clock last night, so I know she didn't get a bath, and I know the night nurse is supposed to do that. It's very frustrating. I felt like he didn't care about her. I can't tell you how much I appreciate you telling me that you do."

"Of course I do. And yes, that is absolutely not a problem. I will change it very soon. I'll change as much of her sheets as I can, too, but I don't want to roll her, because the last time we did, it caused her blood pressure to drop pretty significantly." I remember seeing Brad on my unit this morning. He said he'd be back tonight. "There's a night shift nurse here that I worked with back home. I'll try to get him assigned to your mom, O.K.? I know he'll care just as much as I do. He's good. She'll be in good hands."

She starts crying again. "Thank you so much. I don't want to cause any problems for that other nurse. I'm sure he's great, too. I just haven't been happy with his care the past couple nights, and it's hard to focus on my job when I'm worried about how well he's doing his."

"I completely understand. I was the same way with my Dad. I'll do my best to get my friend assigned to your mom tonight."

"Thank you again, for everything. I'm going to go. I have to work tonight."

It's nearly 1 p.m. She doesn't have much time left to sleep. My heart breaks for her; I was in the same boat with my Dad. I, too, worked nights when he was in and out of the hospital last year. The exhaustion is unreal. "You get some rest," I tell her. "I'll see you tonight."

After she leaves, I tell Kelly I need her to assign my patient to Brad tonight. "And you need to assign Gregory to someone else. He's too much with this patient. Keep her with Richard. I know he's farther away on the unit, but he's much more chill. He's a good combination with her."

"Yeah, that's probably a good idea. I'll do my best tonight. If your friend is assigned to this unit again, I'll give him your assignment."

"Thank you, Kelly. You're the best."

"Well, I do what I can. But you and I need to stop having crazy shifts."

"No kidding."

I check on Gregory. He seems fine. I trust that Richard is still fine and hope that Trisha is still checking in on him regularly. I set to work meticulously cleaning every inch of Gloria's body. I change all her dressings, all her pillowcases, her gown. I organize and label her IV lines, putting all the blood pressure medications together through one lumen of her central line and all the sedation medications together through another lumen. This opens up the third lumen for instant access in case I need to push epi again sometime today. I order the medications from most helpful to least helpful for her current condition. I know this is the best practice now that I've experimented with titrations all morning. She's on Levophed, vasopressin, and phenylephrine. If her blood pressure drops, she responds the quickest to an increase in Levophed. If that doesn't work, an increase in phenylephrine seems to do the trick. She seems least responsive to the vasopressin, so I connect it last. As far as her sedation goes, if her blood pressure is tanking, it's most helpful to pause her paralytic first, so I place it second to her sedative, Versed, on her IV line. I carefully label each line, and then I write down all this information so I can give it to Brad tonight. Each patient is different, and I didn't learn this information from a textbook, but trial and error. I also write down her three-to-one vent settings, and the other vent settings I can remember that caused her blood pressure to drop. I will advise him to try to prevent the residents and respiratory therapists from trying these settings tonight.

I know I shouldn't, but I feel personally responsible for getting Gloria to tomorrow. I desperately don't want to let her daughter down. I saw so much of myself in her eyes. Rationally, I know a lot of my own pain is fueling my thoughts and actions today, but somehow that rational notion doesn't keep me from irrational emotions. I know without a doubt that Gloria isn't going to survive. She should probably have died this morning. But I can't bear to lose her. And I can't bear the thought of leaving her with just any night nurse. I don't trust a nurse who doesn't know me to listen to what I have to say about her medications and ventilator settings. I just need her to make it through my shift. *I* just need to make it through my shift. I'm off tomorrow. Anything can happen to her tomorrow. But I can't handle losing her today.

When I've done everything I can for Gloria, I go to do the same for Gregory. Lucy is in his room tending to her patient, Gregory's roommate. "Hey," she says when I walk in, "can I help you with anything?"

"I should be asking you that. I can't thank you enough for all your help this morning. I seriously don't know what I would've done if you hadn't been in here to take care of Gregory. There was no way I could have left my patient next door."

"I think it's kind of ridiculous that they gave you all these patients. I'm pretty sure you were the only nurse who got tripled today, and you were also the only nurse with patient's sick enough to warrant the crash cart. It's fucked up."

"I agree. I told Kelly not to do this to night shift."

"Good, but they shouldn't have done it to you. Here, let me help you." She takes some bath wipes from me and starts wiping Gregory down on his left side as I continue to clean him on his right. I feel guilty that she's helping me. I have no idea how her day has been, and I know she spent a decent part of it doing my job for Gregory. Before today, we hadn't even met; she didn't have to do that. She didn't owe me anything. I love nurses like Lucy. The only plausible reason for her helping me is that she cared about my patient enough to do it. Not every nurse is like that. Many of them won't do things for patients who aren't assigned to them. They don't see it as their responsibility, even if the life of another nurse's patient is in danger, like Gregory's was today.

We chat as we bathe Gregory and then her patient. I'm thankful that I'm able to help her with something, even if it's small. Lucy tells me that she lives in Brooklyn but is originally from Vermont. She used to be a travel nurse at a different hospital here, but she hasn't worked for the last year or so. Now she's working as a local travel nurse, and her contract ends a few weeks before mine does.

As we're working, someone knocks on the door. We ignore it and they knock again. "Come in!" Lucy shouts over the noise of the negative pressure vent in the corner of the room. Then quietly, to me, she says, "I don't know what the doctor's knocking for. It's not like the patient could have answered if we weren't in here." She rolls her eyes.

I smile; I was thinking the exact same thing. I can tell we're going to be friends.

It feels like an eternity, but the end of the day finally arrives. Kelly tells me that Brad didn't get assigned to return to our unit. I know I'm acting insane, but I have a meltdown over it. "What? Well tell them we need him. I promised the daughter he'd be her nurse tonight!"

"You should know better than to make promises you can't keep to patient's families, Laura."

"I know, but she's really struggling with everything that's been going on, and she wasn't a fan of the nurse who took care of her mom the last couple nights. I can't promise her her mom's life, but I *can* promise her a good nurse. It's all I had to offer her!"

"There are other good nurses here. It's going to be O.K."

"I know, but Kelly, I promised!" I'm nearly shouting at this point and I feel close to tears. "This patient has been trying to die all day, and the only thing that's gotten me through it is knowing I get to give report to a nurse I trust." As I say this, I notice that Gloria's daughter is standing among the night nurses waiting for report. I instantly know that she heard me, and my heart sinks into my stomach.

Kelly sighs. "You have no idea the trouble you're causing, Laura." She picks up the phone and dials the nursing office to request they send Brad here instead of wherever they'd assigned him for the night. I know it's a pain; I thank Kelly profusely and then go over to my patient's daughter.

"Hey!" I tell her, trying to calm myself out of my momentary hysteria. "Don't worry, we're getting the nurse I promised you."

She looks anxious. "I don't want to cause any trouble. The nurse my mom had last night is here. I don't want him to know I was unhappy with him."

"Oh, he won't care," I tell her.

I'm right. He comes up to me after the daughter leaves to go start her own shift and thanks me for getting Gloria assigned to someone else. "She was exhausting last night, and I'm not a fan of the frequent visits of her family."

"No problem," I tell him, happy that this worked out for everyone involved.

Well, everyone except Brad. He looks a little exasperated when he shows up. "What did you do?" he asks me.

"I'm sorry," I tell him. "I didn't think it was going to be a big deal, but I promised this patient's daughter that you'd be her nurse tonight, and then you got assigned to another unit and she showed up to make sure you were her nurse, and I didn't really know what else to do. Sorry."

"They had assigned me to cardiac stepdown. I was only going to have one patient."

"Sorry! If it helps, I did her bath. And your other patient is a potato, so he'll be super easy. And you know you won't get an admission tonight since you're starting out with two instead of one."

"Yeah, whatever. Let me go put my stuff up and then we can do report." He seems annoyed, and reasonably so, but I don't care. I know I'll sleep better tonight knowing that Gloria is in good hands.

I give Brad the reference sheet I made. I have backups for all of her IV medications hanging and ready to go. She still looks clean from the bath I gave her this afternoon. He should be set for the night.

"Someone needs to talk to the family," Brad tells me when I'm done explaining the gravity of our patient's current situation. I shake my head. *He doesn't get it yet.* "There's no point. With COVID, there's no point. No one is willing to let them go."

I wake in the middle of the night in a slight panic from a nightmare in which Gloria died. It takes me a minute to realize it was just a dream. I check the time on my phone: 2 a.m. I try to drift off to sleep again, but I can't seem to relax. My heart is racing from the dream. I reach for my phone again and text Brad to ask how Gloria is doing. He responds about ten minutes later: "Fentanyl's off, Levo and phenyl are down, vent is down from 100% to 80%."

Thank God. Not today. I'm thankful we were able to give that to Gloria's daughter. I can still hear the echoes of her begging God not to take her mother today. Reassured, I drift back to sleep.

*****

I'm not assigned to take care of Gloria when I'm back at work two days later. The nurse who had her on my day off is back today, so she's assigned to her again. I'm bummed, but I know it's probably for the best. I was getting too attached emotionally, and it's only a matter of time before Gloria can no longer be kept alive. I peek in on her first thing in the morning. I ask the nurse how she's been doing.

"Have you had her before?" she asks me.

"Yeah, I took care of her all last week. I talked to her daughter a lot. I've been thinking about her."

"I won't lie to you. It's not looking good. The doctors are going to try to talk to the family again today about withdrawing care."

I'm officially glad I wasn't assigned to care for Gloria today. I don't think I could stomach any more conversations like that with her family. I'm glad I'm here, though, and I let her nurse know I'd be more than happy to help throughout the day if she needs it. My patients that day are all stable, which is why I am able to run in to help when Gloria starts coding.

Somehow, I'm the first one at Gloria's bedside when the monitor nurse calls out that her blood pressure is dropping. I titrate her meds like I did a couple days ago. I grab her hand and tell her it's O.K. That I know she's tired, and her family knows she's tired, and they all love her so very much.

"The family still wants us to code her," a resident tells me as he walks into the room. "So, we're going to do one round of compressions with no meds or ventilation, and then we'll call it."

"O.K. . . . so we're slow coding her?"

"No, we just aren't going to code her for very long."

Jesus Christ. I do not want to be here when that happens.

But just five or ten minutes later, when her heart decides to stop beating, I'm somehow the only one there. I hesitate for a moment, and then I hit the code button. I gently place a sheet over her head to protect myself from COVID particles, tell her I'm sorry for everything she's been through and everything she's about to go through, and remind her how loved she is. I squeezed her hand and promise her I'll be right here the whole time. Then I begin chest compressions.

It all happens in a matter of seconds, but time slows during those moments we are alone. As I compress her heart to keep it beating, I just keep thinking, *Please go, please go, please go.* Her nurse and residents run into the room, but no one does anything. They all just watch me do compressions, and when two minutes is up, one of the residents calls time of death.

"Are you O.K.?" the nurse asks me as I stand there, holding Gloria's hand.

"I'm fine," I say "It's just sad. Want some help making her pretty for the family?"

"That would be great. Thank you. Are you sure you're O.K.?"

"I will be," I say, attempting a smile that most likely doesn't show through all my protective gear.

We work in silence as we turned off all her IV medications and monitors. Disconnect her from everything. Turn off the ventilator. Change her gown, her sheets. Sit her up nicely so that her body looks comfortable. We're paying our respects the only way we know how. It is a strange feeling, to be both happy that someone is no longer suffering and also feel sorrow and grief for those left behind, those left to pick up the pieces. Sadness for the loss that is created by the end of suffering. It is a feeling I'm unwillingly familiar with, both with previous patients and with the loss of my Dad. Every time I've lost a patient since I lost him, I've felt a pang of sorrow for the family of the deceased, because I know that pain is unlike any other. And I know there is nothing, no one, who can save them from the grief that is about to come.

Later in the day, all of Gloria's kids came to say goodbye to her body. The first daughter, one I hadn't met before, yells in sorrow as she weeps. I stand quietly outside the door of the room alongside a couple other nurses who cared for Gloria. As she sobs, I feel tears of my own stinging my eyes. I let a few fall before quickly brushing them away. It's not my place to cry when a family is grieving the loss of a patient of mine. They don't have room for anyone's grief but their own. It's my job to offer them support, hugs, and tissues. I can cry when they leave.

When the oldest daughter emerges from the room, I am ready with a water bottle and a tissue box. I offered my condolences and help her to a chair in the hallway, where we let her catch her breath. The other daughter, the one who works at the hospital, is there in the hallway. She looks stoic. "Hi, Laura," she says quietly.

I again offered condolences and let her know that her mom didn't die alone. I let her sister, weeping in the hallway chair now, know that her mom loved her very much. And now she isn't feeling any pain. And she will always love her and be with her. They both thank me.

And then we all carry on with our day.

THREE MINUTES TOO SOON

I'M TOLD DURING REPORT THAT my patient today, Clara, was transferred to the ICU about an hour before I got here. "She came up from the ED," the night nurse tells me. "She was found down and unresponsive sometime last night. She's in septic shock. Her vitals look O.K. right now, but I had to start an epi drip to keep her heart rate above forty bpm. The Levo and the Neo are on for blood pressure support. If you can titrate any of them down, the docs want the epi drip off, but I honestly don't think that's going to happen today."

"O.K. sounds good," I reply. "Thanks."

"Good news is her daughter made her a DNR last night when the ED doctors explained how sick she is. I'm so thankful. I don't know if I can take another code on a ninety-year-old."

"I know what you mean," I say as I turn to go in to assess Clara.

She looks terrible. Her face and chest appear to be swollen, but upon further inspection I realize they're full of subcutaneous air (air trapped in the tissue just underneath the skin, typically caused by a tear in one or both lungs). I'm grateful she's a DNR. I don't know whether I can handle another futile code either. Her vitals look stable and her drips look full, so I leave to assess my other patient.

The next several hours are fairly smooth as far as vital signs are concerned. There are only a handful of times I have to run into Clara's room to titrate the drips up to higher doses.

At some point in the afternoon, her resident comes to tell me that her daughter has just called. "She wants to let her mother go," he tells me. "She said she can get up here around 3 p.m. Just keep the drips running until then and come find me when she gets here."

"O.K., sounds good," I tell him.

I go into Clara's room and tell her that her daughter will be here soon. I change her gown and sheets so that she looks as presentable as possible, and I take all unnecessary supplies and machines out of the room, replacing them with a chair next to Clara's bedside. I check the drips; they're still pretty full. There's no sense in getting backups if we'll be discontinuing them soon. I look at her vitals; they're stable. I leave the drip rates where they are and go to tend to my other patient.

I'm passing 4 p.m. meds in my other patient's room when I hear the monitor nurse over the radio. "Laura, you need to check on fifty-nine."

I run into Clara's room as fast as I can get a gown on. Her COVID-19 test results aren't back yet, and even though the doctors are pretty sure she'll come back negative, I don't want to take any chances. I see the monitor go from twenty beats per minute to zero in what feels like a fraction of a second. "WHAT?" I scream in disbelief. "NO! Clara, your daughter will be here any minute!"

I draw up two milliliters of epinephrine off her IV drip and slam it into her central line as fast as I can. It doesn't work. I draw up four milliliters, then six, and then ten, slamming each in faster than the next. "JUST HANG ON A FEW MORE MINUTES! SHE'S ON HER WAY!" I'm begging Clara to live, to restart her heart, frantically pushing more and more epi even though I know it's futile. Clara is gone. Her heart stopped minutes ago and no amount of epinephrine will change that. I can't do chest compressions because Clara is a DNR. It's for the best; they wouldn't save her anyway.

I run out to the monitor nurse. "What happened?" I ask her, exasperated.

"I don't know. Her heart rate dropped from sixty to forty in a matter of seconds. By the time you got in there she was flat-lining. There was nothing else to do."

I hear her tell me this, but the words aren't making sense.

"The daughter just called. She's here. I'm going to go down and get her," the resident says, walking up behind us.

I turn, my eyes wide with sorrow and disbelief. "Clara just died," I tell him. "I don't know what happened. I ran in there as soon as I was radioed, but she'd already flat-lined. I pushed epi off her line, but it didn't do anything. I didn't know what else to do. She's just gone." I can hear the hysteria in my voice, but I can't control it.

"It's O.K.," he tells me, placing a hand on my shoulder. "There was nothing else you could have done. I'll talk to the daughter. She knew this could happen."

I don't know what to do. I am beside myself. All I can think is how upset I would be if I had missed my Dad's death by minutes. How robbed I would feel. How hurt I would feel. How unfair it is that Clara died when her daughter was down in the lobby. I go into Clara's room. Aside from the fact that she's dead, she looks presentable. I turn off the monitor, turn off the ventilator, stop all the drips. *I can't be here*, I think. *I can't do this*.

I run down the hall to the other end. I want somebody. Anybody. *Lucy*, I think, *where's Lucy*. I see her pulling meds from the Omnicell at the end of the hall. I half walk, half jog up to her and begin telling her what happened. I'm talking too quickly, and before I know it tears are streaming down my face around my N95. I'm in the middle of the hallway, the middle of the area of the unit with the most traffic. People are looking at me. I'm probably causing a scene. I don't care.

"I tried to push epi, but it didn't work, and I didn't know what else to do," I tell Liz between sobs.

"Oh, honey, it's O.K. You did what you could. It's O.K." Lucy closes the Omnicell and hugs me.

"Laura, what happened?" Ulga says, running up to us.

Through sobs I relay the story again for her.

"Oh Laura, please don't cry! You are such an amazing nurse. If I had to die, I would want you to be my nurse. I would want you beside me. You are the best nurse I've ever met. You truly do everything you can for your patients. Do you remember the last day we worked together? You spent *hours* in that lady's room washing her hair and changing her dressings, and we all knew she was going to die. You did it anyway. That's who I would want to die with if I couldn't have my daughter."

I'm touched by this—Ulga has only worked with me that one time before—but I'm so upset that I can't think to tell her just how much her words mean to me. "But she could have had her daughter," I wail. "She was literally in the lobby. It's not fair. It's just not fair! I failed them both."

"Maybe Clara didn't want her daughter to see her die," Lucy says. "You said you told Clara that her daughter was on her way up, right? Maybe she's like a cat and preferred to die alone. Maybe she could sense that her daughter was downstairs, and that's why she let go. We can't know these things for sure, but some people are just like that. Some hang on for that one person they're waiting to say goodbye to, and others go before their loved ones have a chance to see it happen."

I haven't considered this, even though it's usually something I'm aware of. I've been thinking only about the daughter, who must have wanted to be with Clara when she passed if she was coming up here to see her, to stop the medications and let her go. I am the daughter. I let her down.

My world begins to go dark and fuzzy around the edges, and it occurs to me that I've had my N95 mask on this entire time. I'm still sobbing. "I'm going to go get some water," I tell Lucy and Ulga.

"Sure, I'm here if you need me, O.K.?" Lucy says.

"Thanks," I say. I hurry away to the break room, noticing that the daughter and the resident have arrived to the unit. I feel like I have no right to be this upset in front of her. It's not my mom that just died.

I sit in the break room and focus on slowing my breathing. I feel a numbness shoot through my arms, an identical feeling to the two times panic attacks landed me in the ED the previous year. *I'm O.K. I'm O.K. I'm O.K.,* I think to myself, trying to calm down. *Slow your breathing. Drink your water. It's O.K. I'm O.K.*

I finally get it together enough to go talk to the daughter. I meet her just outside Clara's room. She's coming out. She looks stoic, but not like she's been crying. I hope my mask hides the evidence my meltdown just moments ago. "I am so, so sorry," I say softly to Clara's daughter. "I did everything I could to keep her alive until you got here, but it just wasn't enough."

"I know you did," her daughter says, managing a half-smile. "It's O.K. It was her time. She was ready. It's better this way. She knows I love her."

I am selfishly relieved to hear this. I'm surprised, too—her response so far from how I would have felt if our roles were reversed. She says she's ready to leave, and I silently walk her off the unit. She thanks me at the door—for what, I cannot fathom. I still feel like I have failed her. After she leaves, I look at my watch. 6 p.m. I haven't eaten all day. I ask someone to keep an eye on my other patient. I eat a sandwich, but I cannot taste it. I have no thoughts, just a general feeling of defeat and emptiness.

When I come back out, a couple of the psych nurses are finishing Clara's postmortem care. They've done everything for me. I am overwhelmed with gratitude, and I start to cry again. "Thank you," I tell them. "Thank you so, so much."

"Don't worry about it," one of them says, smiling. "Why don't you just take care of the charting and make sure your other patient doesn't need anything before shift change. We can handle this."

Thank you isn't an adequate phrase, but it's all I have, so I say it again and do as I'm told. I feel depleted. When I get home, I'm so worn out that I sit down for five full minutes in the shower. I have no thoughts. I have no tears. I just feel empty. Inadequate. *What are we doing?* I wonder. *Why can't we save anybody?*

I go to bed.

HAPPY DEATH DAY

CHARLIE, TODAY'S CHARGE NURSE, DOES not share the gratitude of the psychiatric nurse who bought us bagels last week. I can tell he's not a huge fan of travel nurses or being sent to our unit to charge for us, so I'm nervous when I have to ask for his help in setting up my patient's CVVHD machine. "I've never had to set it up before," I explain to him sheepishly. "Back home we had a dialysis nurse who would come do that part for us, and then we'd just monitor and troubleshoot it as it ran."

"Jeez," he scoffs, "are you guys good for anything?" After a slight pause he adds, "I'm just kidding, princess, I'll show you how we do it here in the slums."

The task proves to be more tedious than it is technical. It takes twenty to thirty minutes to completely set up the machine. The problem with this it's twenty to thirty minutes I'm not providing patient care. And unlike back home, these patients are not one-to-one, so I do have more than one patient to care for.

CVVHD machines are notorious for alarming for seemingly no reason. Every time they alarm, they stop cycling blood, which puts the blood at risk for clotting. Not only does the patient lose that volume of blood supply (about 200 to 250 milliliters) but I lose the setup tubing and have to restart the entire process—thirty minutes of machine setup and all. It's a lot easier to catch an alarm early when I'm sitting in the room with the machine rather than in an entirely different room behind a wooden door where I can't hear anything and everyone is too busy to hear the alarm. The charge nurses do try to pair CVVHD patients with less-sick patients, but sometimes that's worse, because patients who are well enough to hit a call light but not well enough to leave the ICU usually expect a lot of attention.

Between me trying to care for my CVVHD patient and the nurse caring for the patient across the hall from him, Charlie is very busy. The patient across the hall is COVID positive, and spends the day desaturating and dropping his blood pressure (which is to say, threatening to die). I feel bad that I can't help, but my hands are full. That afternoon, when I go into the breakroom to eat lunch, I'm met by a tired-looking Charlie.

"I need some coffee," I tell him.

"Yeah, me too. I feel like I can't ever drink enough."

"I know what you mean. I'm the same way."

"Well go get some Starbucks. I'm sure you can afford it. Heck, you could probably afford to buy coffee for the whole unit with how much they're paying you guys to work here." I can tell he's joking, but he's not entirely wrong. "It just sucks," he adds. "We've been busting our butts for weeks trying to help COVID patients without so much as a crisis bonus, and then they fly you guys in here at four to six K a week and most of you just sit on your asses." He quickly looks up at me after saying that and adds, "Not you though. You're fine. You actually work."

"I don't understand anyone who works in the ICU who doesn't expect every shift to be a difficult one. If I wasn't willing to work hard, I certainly wouldn't want to work on this unit."

He smiles at that. "I agree."

On my way back from lunch, I stop to grab a coffee. I grab one for Charlie, too. I understand what he was saying, and I know he's been crazy busy helping me and the nurse across from me. I like to think it softened him to us a little. By 6 p.m., my CVVHD machine has completely clotted off for the second time this shift. Charlie tells me to just get the supplies ready and have night shift set it up so that I have time to get meds passed for both my patients before shift change. I'm relieved.

Not long after I've finished this task, I hear the nurse across the hall yell for the crash cart. I rush it into her room and find a crowd of residents around the patient's bed. The nurse is trying to explain to them all that has happened throughout her shift. I can see that there aren't any other nurses in the room, so I get ready to do compressions. I cover the patient's head with a pillowcase to protect us all from the expulsion of COVID particles that happens when chest compressions are performed, place the AED pads on his chest, and get the bed lowered to a position in which I can effectively push on his chest. I've just barely placed my hands in the correct position on his chest when I see a flatline on his monitor. I begin compressions. About a minute in, my eye shield falls off my face and onto the bed. *Oh well.* I ask someone to get me a mask with a shield on it. Some of the male residents keep asking whether I need a break, but I ignore them. I'm fine for my full round of two minutes.

There are two rounds after mine until we get a pulse back. I can't help but notice that no one asks the men whether they need relief from giving compressions. I mosey my way on over to the other side of the bed, where the patient's IV medications are hanging. They're a mess. I don't know what's what or where it's going or where to push new meds. I become fixated on organizing them. I'm halfway done when a nurse pops her head into the room and says, "Hey, we need some of you guys in room thirty-eight. She's coding, too."

"*Shit*," I hear the fellow say under his breath as he runs out of the room.

We keep coding this guy for an hour. I alternate between giving compressions and pushing meds. There's one female resident in the room. When she steps up to do a round of compressions, she is met with the same remarks I got: "Let us know if you need to stop."

I roll my eyes and raise my voice to tell her, "I don't hear them saying that to the boys, do you? But if you ask me, we're getting the prettiest wavelengths on the monitor."

She smiles at me and keeps going. We code him for the last hour, maybe hour and a half, of our day. When night shift arrives to take over, I hear that the other patient has been coding that entire time, too, taking nearly all the staff off the floor to run these two codes. It's going to be a long night, but both patients are still alive by the time I clock out.

Another shift a few days later proves to be just as grim. I learn that both of the patients we coded during my last shift are still alive, but one of them was moved to Main ICU for closer monitoring, and the other one is currently existing at an oxygen saturation of 60%. I find this infuriating. "And they don't want to palliatively extubate him? He's basically suffocating to death through a straw."

"I know," replies his nurse for the day, a grim look on her face, "but apparently family won't agree to it."

"Did they explain that we're essentially torturing him by letting him exist like this?"

She shakes her head. Of course they have. And of course family doesn't understand. They seldom do. And the physicians aren't going to force them to unplug their loved one. But they should. This is a cruel way to go, and anyone in healthcare would agree he's currently more dead than alive.

I'm glad he is not my patient. I don't have it in me to be placed in situations like that right now. It's both sad and enraging. Everyone thinks the hardest part of being an ICU or ER nurse is watching people die, but it's not. The hard part is watching people suffer. The hard part is trying to explain to grieving friends and family members that what we're doing is hurting them more than it is helping. The hard part is arguing with physicians that what they're asking us to do to a patient is inhumane but having to do it anyways because legally it's not our call to make. The hard part is watching patients gasp for air through a ventilator tube that's been in place way longer than it should've been as they slowly, slowly, reach for death across the span of twelve to forty-eight hours. The hard part is knowing that you're probably hurting more than you're helping but that you have to do it anyways. The hard part is wondering whether there was something we could've done that we didn't do before the patient got to this point. The hard part is holding the hand of someone who's dying alone, fear in their eyes, wondering what they're thinking and trying to say something meaningful, but not knowing what to say. The hard part is going home at night after a long fourteen-hour shift wondering whether you even made the slightest difference. The hard part is constantly apologizing—to patients, physicians, family members, other nurses—for things that aren't you fault and that you can't fix, but that you're sorry for anyway.

"I'm sorry your mom is dying, but there's nothing else we can do."

"I'm sorry you're in pain, but I can't give you any more medication."

"I'm sorry I haven't given that medication yet. I've been stuck in another patient's room. A patient who is sicker than this one."

"I'm sorry I haven't had a chance to tend to this patient yet."

"I'm sorry there are no visitors allowed right now. I'm sure that's very frustrating."

"I'm sorry your bed is uncomfortable."

"I'm sorry the food isn't any good."

"I'm sorry I didn't come the minute you hit your call light. I was trying to save a different patient's life."

"I'm sorry we've kept you alive this long with no improvement."

"I'm sorry there's a gaping wound on your ass because you aren't able to move or turn yourself in bed."

"I'm sorry I'm exhausted and overwhelmed and unable to use a perfect customer service–style voice and etiquette with you right now."

"I'm sorry the news I'm giving you isn't what you wanted to hear."

"I'm sorry you're going through this right now."

I'm sorry, I'm sorry, I'm sorry. The list goes on and on. And I truly am so, so sorry—for all of it—but there's only so much I can do.

*****

We lose the patient. By the end of the shift, we've lost three more, all due to COVID-19.

HIS NAME IS RICHARD

I HAVE AVOIDED BEING ASSIGNED to Richard for weeks. (Remember Richard? The potato I took care of during week one? When I had three patients?) Each day his nurse is increasingly frustrated by the physicians' lack of willingness to do anything for him. "He's just rotting away in there, and nobody seems to care," I hear her say.

I'm really glad that it's not my problem.

In nursing interviews, I used to always emphasize that I don't believe in the phrases like "That's not my patient," "That's not my job," or "That's not my problem." "If it's a patient in my hospital, it's my problem!" I'd say with a smile on my face. I've let go of a lot of things I used to say and do. I'm doing my best just to survive the current circumstances and ensure my patients do as well.

I'm not entirely sure what happens with Richard throughout the shift. My patients are in the two rooms across the hall from him, and they're very sick, so I'm busy most of the morning. At some point, Richard's nurse tells me that his wife and mother-in-law are coming up to say goodbye before they finally let him go.

"Took them long enough," I say. Poor Richard has been more dead than alive for weeks.

When Richard's wife walks onto the unit, I can see that she's already crying, accompanied by his somber-looking mother-in-law. His nurse is in another patient's room, so I gown up to go in, just in case the residents or Richard's wife need anything. When she walks into the room, she lets out a soul-crushing wail. "My Richard! Oh, my baby," she exclaims. She is sobbing now, standing at the head of his bed, looking at him. There are two residents and a fellow in Richard's room. Even under their masks, I can tell by their expressions that they're not sure what to do. I want to go to Richard's wife and put a hand on her back, but the room is too small for me to navigate over next to her. I ask the fellow whether there's anything I can do.

"Go override two milligrams of versed, please," he tells me.

I come back with the medication. I explain what it's for as I push it, but through her tears, I don't think Richard's wife can hear me. Mentally, she is probably on another planet right now. She pulls out her phone, and I'm afraid I'm going to have to tell her that photographs of patients or the facility are not allowed when she turns the phone around to face us. The screen displays a picture of a man. "This is my Richard," she screams through her sobs. "He is a person! Do you see him? DO YOU SEE HIM?" she yells at no one in particular, shaking her phone in the air. "He was the love of my life! He was a person. To you people he is just a body in a bed, but he was a PERSON. Oh my Richard!"

She puts the phone away and turns her attention back to her husband. She begins to stroke his feet with her gloved hands as she sobs, repeating "My Richard, my Richard!" over and over again. I remember referring to him as a potato the last time I was his nurse. I hate myself. I say something lame like, "Of course he was. And he is so lucky to have a loving wife like you."

The fellow seems at a loss for words, other than, "I'm so sorry, ma'am. We did everything we could."

Richard's wife doesn't care. She isn't listening. She isn't here.

Eventually, Richard takes his last breath. His mother-in-law comes out into the hallway, sits on the couch. I hand her a box of tissues and a water bottle. "It's O.K. to take your mask off out here for a minute," I tell her. "I don't want you to hyperventilate." I'm speaking from my experience the other day after I lost Clara.

"I'm alright, dear, but thank you." She forces a small smile onto her face. "I don't think I can say the same for my daughter, though. Someone should tell her that when she comes out."

"Of course," I say.

I go back by the nursing monitors to peek in on Richard's wife. She has her gloves and mask off now, and she is kissing his face.

"Someone should stop her," I say, alarmed. "In addition to COVID, he has some sort of terrible killer bug. It's highly contagious! Why aren't the doctors getting her out of there?"

"Let her be. She's grieving." Casey says.

"I know, but she'll be our next patient if someone doesn't stop her."

"She's been told the risks," Casey says. "What else can we do?"

That's a good question. What can we do? I have a feeling Richard's wife's answer would be: Not enough.

THIRTEEN DRIPS AND A GI BLEED

THE NEXT MORNING, I WAKE up to a text from Maddi. There's a link to a news clip and a text that reads, *Be careful babe. This was in Brooklyn.*

I click on it and soon I'm watching a large crowd of people standing around what appears to be a police car. The man filming begins to narrate: "We are here in downtown Brooklyn, where a crowd of protestors was just run down by this police car. The crowd is not happy about this." Behind him, the car begins to rock back and forth. People are pushing it on either side, making it sway. "A few people were hit by this car, which has since been abandoned by the police."

"FUCK YOU, PIGS!" someone shouts in the background as a Molotov cocktail flies in the air.

"Woah!" the camera man shouts as he ducks. "People are really angry. Someone just threw what I can only assume is a Molotov cocktail at the abandoned police car. Babe, we should get back. That thing could blow." He and his companion move back, and he continues to narrate as people in the crowd shout things like "Fuck you, pigs!" and "Fuck NYPD!" in the background. Eventually, the police car blows up.

Tears sting my eyes as I watch. I wonder whether anyone got hurt. I wonder whether any of the hospitals can handle an influx of trauma patients right now. Our makeshift ICU is still full of COVID patients. *What is happening to the world?* I check the time. 5:20. *Dang it.* It's an hour before my usual wake-up time for work. After watching that video, I have too many thoughts and emotions to fall back to sleep.

I decide to deal with these emotions the same way I've been dealing with all the other ones I've accumulated in New York: I go for a run. I have time for only two miles, but it's two more than I had planned for so I consider it an accomplishment. I feel better when I get back home. My head feels clearer. For once, I have time to make breakfast and pack a lunch before my shift. I eat scrambled eggs and toast. I sip my coffee. I go to work.

The minute I get there I'm thankful for my morning run and my breakfast. I've been assigned to care for one of our long-time COVID patients, Marcus. Marcus has been here for nearly two months, and early this morning he began to take a turn for the worse. "He's got a fever of 107," the night nurse tells me. "I've given him Tylenol. I've got him sandwiched between two cooling blankets. I've put ice all over him. I don't know what else to do. It won't come down."

"O.K.," I say. I go into his room. There are three different IV poles with one, two, three . . . ten different IV drips hanging. He's intubated and receiving tube feeds, and there are two cooling blanket machines next to his bed. The room is hardly big enough for all this equipment, and the bed is hardly big enough for this nearly 300-pound patient. I take a deep breath. It's going to be a long day.

"Hello love!" Arina says in a sing-song voice as she comes into the room. "I get to work with you today!"

Thank God. I breathe a sigh of relief. I've worked with Arina as my helper nurse for several shifts now. We work very efficiently together, and we've begun to develop a close friendship.

"Woah!" she says, taking a look at all the IV medications. "That's a lot of drips."

"I know, and he has a fever of 107. They've given him Tylenol, cooling blankets, ice packs. None of it is working."

"I'll get more ice packs. It can't hurt anything."

"Good idea. Thanks." I walk into the resident's room to see whether the day shift resident, Jake, has any ideas the night shift one didn't.

"We can try IV Tylenol, but after that I'm out of ideas," Jake tells me.

"Good idea. I hadn't thought of that," I reply. I try to remember whether I've ever even given IV Tylenol. I can't say that I have. I call pharmacy and ask them to send it as soon as they can. "He has a fever of 107," I tell them.

"O.K., we'll have it tubed up in ten or fifteen minutes."

"Did I just hear you say 107?" Kelly asks me.

"Yeah, it's Marcus."

"Dang, he's really not doing well today. Let me know if you need any help."

"Thanks. I will." I'm glad Kelly is the charge nurse today. I don't know how she always manages to work on days I'm fighting the biggest fires, but I'm grateful for it. I know she'll be there when I need her.

One of the other nurses on the unit also overheard Marcus's temperature, and he tells me he's pretty sure the record for highest fever ever in a live human is 108. *That can't be good.* I wonder whether he's right, but I don't have time to check.

I've just finished hanging the IV Tylenol (drip number eleven) when Jake walks into the room. "Hey," he says, "I just saw Marcus's lab work. I don't know why, but his hemoglobin is dropping. Six-point-two. We're going to have to give him blood."

"Of course we are," I reply. "Thanks for letting me know. I'll get right on it." IV drip number twelve.

Nearly an hour later, I hear the monitor nurse over the radio. "Laura, your patient's blood pressure is dropping. Seventy-nine over forty."

Shit. He's on all four blood pressure support medications that exist; we don't have any more. I go to check on him. The blood transfusion is almost finished. None of the IV drips are running low. I titrate them up, but now I'm maxed out on all four. Past that, there's nothing I can do.

Jake comes into the room. "What the hell is going on with this guy?" he asks no one in particular.

"I wish I knew," I tell him.

"How much room do you have on the phenylephrine?"

"None," I say sadly, "I just maxed it out."

"Damn it. And the blood is finished?"

"Just about. We could push fluids?" I offer.

"Yeah, let's do it. I don't know what else to try. I really need this guy to make it."

I make a face. Marcus is closer to dead than alive right now.

"I know he's in bad shape," Jake says, as if he can read my mind, "but he was doing so well. He's the only COVID patient I've had who is still alive. I've been here since March and I haven't saved a single person. He's young, I thought he could be my save. He's been my beacon of hope this past month. I feel like such a failure."

I am deeply saddened by Jake's words. I know exactly how he feels, and I have no idea how to comfort him.

"Try the fluids," he says. "Push as much as you need to in order to stabilize his blood pressure. Radio me if you need me, and if you can think of any other ideas, please let me know. I'm at a loss."

I pop my head out of the room to ask Anna for supplies. "Grab me a few bags of LR, some gravity tubing, and a couple of pressure bags."

"O.K.!"

Marcus's blood pressure is still dropping. I need to do something, and fast. I titrate one of the blood pressure medications slightly above the max to hold his pressure steady until I can get the fluids. Soon, Arina comes in with the supplies. "Here's the LR and some gravity tubing, but I can't find any pressure bags. Kelly is looking for us, but I figured we should get these going."

I sigh. "Of course. All right, I'll just push it myself until she gets here." I think back to Imani. Although she didn't have COVID, she *did* have an extremely low blood pressure that the fellow and I were able to stabilize by hand-pushing several bags of LR and a few ampules of bicarb. "Hey Jake," I radio as I begin to squeeze a bag of LR into Marcus's IV, "can we try bicarb? I'll be honest, I haven't seen his latest ABG, but at this point I don't think it could hurt anything."

"Good idea," he radios back. "I'll put in an order for an ampule and a new ABG. Are the fluids helping?"

"Not yet. I'll keep pushing them."

I send Arina down to pharmacy to grab the bicarb, it'll be faster than waiting for them to bullet it up. Kelly comes into the room with a handful of tongue depressors and tourniquets. "I can't find any pressure bags," she tells me, "but I thought we could make one."

"With popsicle sticks?" I ask in disbelief.

"Technically," she scoffs back, "these are tongue depressors. And yes. Don't doubt me." Kelly and I have a shared sarcasm and dark sense of humor. Bantering with each other often helps relieve the tension of the stressful situations we always seem to find ourselves dealing with together.

I keep hand-pushing the fluids while Kelly tapes several tongue depressors together. She spikes another bag of LR, hangs it, and wraps the tongue depressors around the bag. "O.K.," she tells me, "stop doing that for a second and hold these things in place." I do as she says, still wondering how this is going to resemble anything close to a pressure bag. She ties several tourniquets around the tongue depressors, and I start to see fluid pouring into the drip chamber of the IV line. "There," she says proudly, "just like a pressure bag. Don't ever doubt my abilities."

"I wouldn't dream of it," I laugh. This make-shift pressure bag frees me to do other things. I've never been so grateful for tongue depressors.

Arina arrives with the bicarb, and when I push it, Marcus's blood pressure rises almost immediately. *Yes.* "Hey Jake," I radio, "The bicarb helped. I think you should order a drip."

"I'll order one, but I'll need that ABG. Pharmacy won't verify my order without it."

I ask Arina to grab the ABG so I can switch out the fluids for a new bag, thankful that she asked me to teach her how to do that out of boredom earlier this week. The next hour feels chaotic. I am frantically switching out IV bags that are running dry and hanging fresh bags of fluid. It takes a lot of effort to manage to tie Kelly's make-shift pressure bag system onto a new bag of fluids by myself, and the longer it takes me, the lower Marcus's blood pressure drops. Doctors and respiratory therapists continually pop into the room as I work, asking me and each other questions, trying to come up with other things to try.

We are essentially treating Marcus with trial and error at this point. The fluids are helping, so we keep giving them. A change in his ventilator settings doesn't help anything, so we change them back. His temperature is 106 after receiving the IV Tylenol, and we can't give him any more for the next twenty-four hours without killing his liver. According to his lab work, and indicated by his lack of urine, his kidneys aren't doing very well, but we can't start dialysis when he's this unstable. "If we can't get his temperature down, he's probably going to code," the attending says. "His body just can't tolerate it."

I take a deep breath. What else can we do? Then it hits me. "The Arctic Sun!" I exclaim. *Why didn't I think of this sooner?* "Do we have an Arctic Sun?"

The physicians look confused.

"Yeah, the Arctic Sun!" I say again. "We use it to cool people after ROSC"—return of spontaneous circulation, or the return of a pulse during a code— "to prevent brain damage. I don't see why we couldn't use it to cool him down from his fever."

"I don't know whether we have that or not," the attending tells me.

Surely we do. This is a trauma hospital. "Kelly," I radio, "do we have an Arctic Sun?"

"The ICU does," she radio's back. "I'll have to see if it's available. Why?"

"We want to use it to try to get Marcus's fever down," I tell her. "I can't believe I didn't think of it sooner."

"Oh, good idea! I'll run down and grab it."

This feels like the first victory I've had all day.

Arina comes in with the bicarb drip (IV drip number thirteen), and after it's been infusing for a while, Marcus's blood pressure starts to stabilize. *Thank goodness.* Kelly comes in with the Arctic Sun. "Don't hate me," she says tentatively, "but I'm going to have to give you another patient. You're the only nurse left with only one. I think it'll be a couple hours before she gets here, so you'll have time to grab something to eat first. Hopefully Marcus will stay stable long enough for us to get her settled."

I groan at the idea. I was just beginning to feel like I could catch my breath.

When I come back from lunch, Kelly is halfway through setting up a CVVHD machine in Marcus's room.

"They want to start dialysis?" I ask in disbelief. "This morning they agreed with me that he's too unstable."

"Yeah," Kelly answers as she works, "but he's been good ever since we started the bicarb, so now they want to try it. He hasn't produced any urine in the last couple days, and his potassium levels are starting to get too high." Patients with potassium levels of greater than five are at higher risk for lethal dysrhythmias—the heart rhythms that cause code blues. "Don't worry, I've done the hard part of setting the machine up, and I told the ED they'll have to hold your admission until we get this up and running."

"O.K.. Thanks, Kelly."

I take over the rest of the CVVHD setup. I've just barely gotten it running when my admission shows up. I turn to leave Marcus's room and help settle my new patient next door when the machine starts alarming. Shoot. "Anna, can you get her hooked up to the monitor? I'll be there as soon as I fix this."

"I'm on it."

I troubleshoot the machine as best I can, but at times they can be very temperamental, and it looks like this is going to be one of those times. I ask another nurse on the unit whether she can keep troubleshooting it for me long enough to keep the blood from clotting while I do a quick assessment of my admission.

The admission's name is Kate. When I enter her room, she's crying. Arina is doing her best to soothe her as she gets her hooked up to the monitors. *Lord help me.* I fear I'm too stressed to be a calming presence for my patient. I do my best to smile through my mask instead of crazy eyes and force a cheery tone. "Hi Kate! I'm Laura, and I'll be your nurse today."

"Hi," she says through tears.

"Kate, can you tell me a little bit about what's going on? What brought you into the hospital today?"

"Well, I went to the bathroom at work, and when I looked in the toilet, it was full of blood. As the day has gone on, I've gotten increasingly dizzy. After the second bloody bowel movement, I came to the emergency room. They said I'm going to need surgery? I've never been in the hospital before!"

"Not necessarily surgery, but you will need to have a rectal scope done so the doctors can find and stop the bleeding."

This doesn't seem to reassure her at all. "I don't want to die!" she says, starting to cry again. She looks down as she says this, and when she does, I give Arina a look that I pray she understands as *help me.*

"Don't worry," Arina jumps in immediately. "We are going to take very good care of you. Just because you are in the ICU doesn't mean you're going to die. It just means that there is potential for your condition to worsen, so your physicians wanted to have you with the best nurses possible. But your vital signs are stable right now, and we're giving you blood to replace what you're losing in your stool. You're safe here, we'll take care of you." This seems to calm Kate down a little. I am very thankful for Anna's background in psychiatry.

Kate tells us she needs a bedpan. On my way to go get her one, I hear the CVVHD machine alarming from inside Marcus's room. Dang it. I pop in there, troubleshoot it a couple times, and return to getting the bedpan. On my way out of the supply room, I pass the nurse who helped troubleshoot the CVVHD machine earlier. "Hey," she says when she sees me, "I think I fixed it, but I'm honestly not sure why it was alarming."

"Yeah, I'm not sure either," reply. "It's yelling at me again."

"Oh no. I'll come help you take a look at it just as soon as I give my patient her pain medicine."

"Thanks. No rush," I tell her as I hurry on back to Kate's room. I feel bad. I know everyone else is busy, too.

I took too long with the bedpan; Kate has gone in the bed. Now instead of crying about her fears of dying, she's crying of embarrassment. "I'm so sorry!" she tells me when I see the mess. "I've never done that before in my life!"

"Don't be sorry," I say immediately. "You've never had a GI bleed before, either. You can't help it, honey. I know it's embarrassing to you, but I promise I see this type of thing all the time. It's not a big deal to me, and it's an easy fix. Let me just run and grab some fresh sheets."

I hear the CVVHD machine alarming again when I go back out into the hall. I troubleshoot the alarm, grab some sheets and bath wipes, and head back into Kate's room. Arina and I instruct her on how to roll so that we can change the sheets with her in the bed. I am thankful, at least, that Kate can do the rolling herself. I explain to her that, because of the amount of blood-loss she's experiencing, I don't want her to get up. Anna told me that Kate's pressure dropped pretty low when she had had the bowel movement. "It could cause a sudden drop in your blood pressure," I tell Kate.

We've just barely buttoned the last button on Kate's new gown when she begins to cry again. "I need the bedpan! I don't understand why this is happening. I just want it to stop!"

I try not to look as frazzled as I feel. I would never tell Kate this, but I want it to stop just as badly as she does. Arina and I try to console her some more as we put her on the bedpan. I'm getting worried about the CVVHD machine. I still haven't figured out the cause of the alarm; I've just been giving the machine Band-Aid fixes to keep Marcus's blood moving. A CVVHD machine holds about 210 milliliters of blood when it is circulating. Every time the machine alarms, the blood sits still. The longer the blood sits still, the higher the chances that it will clot in the machine. And if that happens, I'll be unable to return the blood from the machine back to Marcus's body. I know, based on the high amounts of blood pressure medications Marcus is on, and from the three liters of LR that I had to give him this morning, that Marcus can't afford to lose the equivalent of half a unit of blood right now.

I tell Arina I'm going to try to figure out the cause for the CVVHD alarms again, but that I'll be back soon so I can help her get Kate off the bedpan. Sure enough, when I enter Marcus's room, the machine is alarming again. I try every suggestion displayed on the machine's screen for possible solutions, but nothing works. When I get a closer look at the blood that should be circulating, I can see that it's beginning to clot. *This is why these patients need to be one-to-one. Fuck it.*

I decide to return the blood. Dialysis for Marcus is going to have to wait until my admission is more stable. The monitor tech has radioed me twice since I came in here to tell me that Kate's blood pressure is consistently dropping. I trust that if Anna didn't think she could handle the situation for the few minutes I said I would be gone, she would come get me, so I take the extra few minutes in Marcus's room to return the blood and discontinue the CVVHD. Taking Marcus off dialysis isn't going to kill him immediately, but the loss of 210 milliliters of blood might, and it is just physically impossible for me to spend this much time in his room right now. It's the type of nursing judgement I hate having to make. The nursing license exam is full of scenarios like this. *All these things are important, and you must complete each task, but which task is the* most *important? Which one must you do* right now? Right now, I know I must stabilize Kate.

I head back into her room. Her blood pressure is around sixty over forty, and she looks like she might faint any second. "Kate? Kate, can you hear me?!" I ask her, trying not to sound panicked.

"Mhmm."

"I need a resident to room fifty-two. *Now.*"

I increase the rate on both Kate's fluids and her blood transfusion. The faster we can replace the volume of blood she's losing via stool, the better. I promised her she wouldn't die.

"What is it?" a female resident asks me as she enters Kate's room.

"Her blood pressure is dropping. I think she's losing blood faster than we're replacing it. I'm pushing fluids, but we're going to need more blood. Can you order a CBC and a couple fluid boluses of LR?"

The resident looks skeptical. "Sure," she says, and leaves the room. At this point in my nursing career, I've learned that if I remain the most confident and calm person in the room, everyone else will follow suit. I keep pushing fluids. Kate comes to.

"I don't feel so good," she says to no one in particular. Arina looks worried.

I do my best to soothe them both. "It's O.K., we've got you," I tell Kate, grabbing her hand. "We're going to give you more blood. Everything is going to be O.K." I have no right to say this; I have no idea how things are going to be. Kate's blood pressure comes up as she begins to cry again.

"Oh God!" she cries. "I did it again."

"Yes," I say, too happy that her blood pressure is rising to care that she's in distress, "but it's O.K. Your blood pressure is coming back up. I'm right here. I've got you. We've got you. Take some deep breaths for me."

I'm instructing Kate to breathe in and breathe out when, over the radio, the monitor tech calls for me. "Laura," she says, the tension palpable in her voice, "you need to check on Marcus." My heart drops into my stomach. I shoot a panicked glance at Arina, who nods and takes over the deep breathing exercise with Kate.

A female resident meets me in Marcus's room. His blood pressure is plummeting. *What in the world?* My eyes are scanning the IV pumps as fast as they can, trying to find the drip among the thirteen that's beeping to tell me it's empty. I don't hear any beeping and I can't see any blinking lights. It doesn't make any sense. "OH MY GOD," the resident yells, causing me to jump. She's standing next to the ventilator, looking panicked. "THE FUCKING VENTILATOR IS OFF!"

"*What?*" I don't understand. How could the ventilator be *off?* Marcus's blood pressure is the problem, not his oxygenation. I glance at the monitor and notice that his oxygen saturation is starting to trend down, too. I glance at the ventilator. It is, in fact, off. *Fuck.* "HOW THE FUCK DO YOU TURN THIS THING ON?" the resident screams.

"I need respiratory therapy to room forty-two!" I scream into the radio. "NOW! IT'S AN EMERGENCY. I don't know how, but this ventilator is OFF!" I join the resident in her frantic search for an ON button. We find one just as an army of medical staff comes running into the room.

"It's O.K.," the resident says, sighing in relief as she takes a look around. "We fixed it. Somehow this ventilator got put on standby."

"How the *fuck* does that happen?" the attending asks the room. No one answers. I certainly don't know. I'm trying to get my heart rate down. "You have to push *three* buttons to put a ventilator on standby. So, someone please tell me how the fuck that happened on accident?" He looks around the room again. Everyone remains silent. The female resident and I are breathing heavily, like we've just finished running a marathon. Everyone else avoids eye contact. I didn't even know ventilators *had* a standby setting, let alone know how to use it.

"Laura?" he looks at me. "Do you need anything?"

I look at the monitor. Marcus's vitals are stable. "No," I say tentatively. "I think we're O.K." Slowly, the other residents begin to back out of the room.

Eventually, it's just the female resident and I left standing. Jake must be on break. "Phew!" she says. "I thought we were going to have to code him."

"Let's hope we don't," I reply. I take another look at the monitor; vitals are still stable. My eyes gloss over the thirteen

IV drips; none of the bags look less than half empty. I decide it's safe to go back to Kate's room.

When I walk in, Kate's resident is talking rapidly to Kelly. "We'll have to do the massive transfusion protocol. She's losing blood too quickly. I'm going to call the O.R. and let them know she needs to be seen right away." *That's not good.*

"I'll go down to the ICU and get the massive transfuser," Kelly says. "Anna, you go to blood bank and get the cooler."

I guess I'll stay here with Kate I think She looks like she's been dozing in and out of consciousness for a while now.

Some confusion follows as to whether or not we're actually going to do the massive transfusion protocol. Apparently, the day shift resident ordered it right before the night shift resident came on, and he didn't think it was necessary. I let Kelly figure it out while I try to get the CVVHD machine in Marcus's room ready to go for night shift.

Night shift shows up at about the same time that Anna comes back with the cooler of blood products. She and Kelly get the blood running into Kate's IV while I give a hurried report to the night shift nurse taking over for Marcus. "I'm really sorry," I start out, "but today has been super hectic. His temperature was 107 at the beginning of my shift, which is why we have the Arctic Sun on him. And at some point his ventilator got put on standby. And I tried to start CVVHD for a couple hours, but my new admit next door was so unstable I eventually just had to give up. I've been trying to get it set up so that all you have to do is start it, but there hasn't been much time." I take a deep breath. The speed of my speech matches my heart rate. I can feel my heart pounding in my chest.

"Don't worry about it," the night-shift nurse says, looking around the room, which is a complete mess. "I've had him before. I'll figure it out. You go see what they need next door. I'll be fine."

"O.K.," I say uncertainly. "Thanks for understanding. I'm really sorry again!" I've never left a patient's room in such disarray before. I remind myself that I didn't really have a choice.

When I walk into Kate's room, it's in total chaos. Kelly and the night nurse are frantically hanging bag after bag of blood products as Arina scans them into the computer. I'm never going to be able to give report. I desperately need to get out of here.

To my surprise, the night-shift nurse taking over Kate tells me to go ahead and start giving her report while she works. I've gone over all the information I have except for the location of Kate's IVs when Kelly asks the night nurse to help her with something. *So close.* I don't think I could help any more if I tried. Kelly is asking her something about the blood products, something about how the order doesn't match what she's scanning, and I impatiently wait for them to figure it out. I'm half-tempted to just leave; she'll find the IVs. But I'm worried she might have questions or expect me to do something else for Kate before I leave, so I wait.

Thankfully, she has no further questions or requests. I leave quickly before she has a chance to change her mind. I feel bad that Kelly is staying late to help when I'm not, but I remind myself that she's the charge nurse. It's her job to make sure the unit doesn't drown. My job is just to care for my patients until the next shift takes over. I'm leaving a mess behind, but I've done my job.

Arina is waiting for me outside the unit doors. She's laughing. "Have you ever left such a big mess behind in your entire career?"

"No." I begin to laugh too. It's good medicine after a day like today. "I truly can't say that I have!" We go back to my place and kill a bottle of wine as we relive the day with a mixture of disbelief and thank-God-that's-over-and-everybody's-alive. I'm grateful I don't have to work tomorrow.

A NOT-SO-HAPPY BIRTHDAY TO ME

THE NUMBER OF PROTESTS THAT turn into riots in the city begins to increase. Actually, it's happening all over the world. Every morning, the news is showing more and more videos like the one Maddi sent me of people burning down police cars, looting shops in downtown Manhattan, and vandalizing police departments. My landlord messages me to ask whether I'm O.K. and to advise me against going anywhere alone, especially at night, until things quiet down. I appreciate her checking in on me. It's the type of thing my mom would do, and I find it comforting.

A few days into the chaos, Governor Cuomo decides to instate an 8 p.m. city-wide curfew. It will begin tonight, on June 1, and last through the end of the week. My birthday is in two days, and Anna had planned for a social distanced party in the park for me. I realize, sadly, that this will no longer be an option.

My birthday comes, and a slight twinge of sadness is tugging at me from the moment my alarm goes off. I can't remember the last time I had to work on my birthday. Being an only child, and somewhat of a miracle baby at that (my parents tried for over fifteen years to conceive me), my birthday had been a big deal my entire life. Unsurprisingly, the first person to text me happy birthday is Ally, followed a few minutes later by Arina. When I arrive at work, I'm told that I will be the monitor nurse. Fuck yes. I might be at work, but all I really have to do is sit, listen for alarms on the tele monitor, and walkie concerning alarms to other nurses. Happy birthday to me.

I wait all morning for a text from Jake, which eventually comes mid-morning, as does a text from my mom. Facebook posts occasionally pop up wishing me a happy birthday, although I feel like there are less this year than normal. Maybe it's because I'm watching for their arrival all day. After lunch, I take a picture of myself in COVID PPE with "happy birthday to me" written on the front of the protective gown. I post it with a comment that says I'm glad to be working, but it isn't entirely true. In some sense, I am glad, because working is much less depressing than sitting alone in my Airbnb would have been, but it's still depressing. What's worse, none of the friends I've made at the hospital seem to be working today. The day feels long and lonely. One of them was originally going to come over this evening, but with the riot curfew they'd have no way to get home.

I have no plans. I have no presents. I have no cake. I was going to buy myself one on my way home, but with the new curfew I don't have time. This is twenty-five. The sadness takes over the minute I opened my Airbnb's mailbox: it's completely empty. My mom sent me a card a few days early, but I haven't received cards from anyone else, and no one has sent me a gift (I'll get boxes from two of my best friends back home a couple days after my birthday). I was hoping my gift from Jake would be in the mail when I got home (hopefully accompanied by a much-needed love note), but there's nothing. I burst into tears almost the minute I open my front door. I try to get a grip in the shower. I feel so depleted that I sit on the floor and let warm water run over me for who knows how long.

Once I'm out and dried off, I pour myself a glass of birthday whiskey (at least I bought *myself* a present) and call Jake.

"Hey babe, happy birthday. How was your day?"

I burst into tears. "Honestly it was fine, I didn't even have to take patients, but none of my friends were working, and I didn't have any mail waiting for me when I got home, and I just can't stop crying."

"O.K." He's quiet for a moment. "Well, I told you I sent a gift the other day. It should be there by tomorrow."

"I know, Jake, it's not about the present. I'm just sad and it's been a lonely day."

He sounds hostile when he speaks, and the words I hear in his silences are, *You* chose *to be in New York on your birthday. This is no one's doing but your own.* As if it's too much to ask my husband to freaking give a shit that I spent my first birthday without my Dad at work, alone, 1,209 miles from home and everyone I love. As if needing his sympathy in this moment is me asking for too much.

And as if it's *hard* to ship a birthday present early enough for it to arrive either early or on time for the actual date of my birthday. He's only known that my birthday was on June 3 and that I'd be spending it alone in New York since April 17. Apparently, two months is not enough time to purchase a fucking present. Apparently, that's too much to ask of my own husband. I don't need anything material, or for him to spend money on me. A few weeks ago, I was very insistent and sincere when I said over the phone that all I wanted was a heart-felt card I could read when I got home from work today. How hard is that?

I don't want to fight on my birthday—I expected Jake to make me feel better, not worse—so I tell him I have to go because I work tomorrow, too. Our tones are tense when we hang up, and we've barely talked to each other, but I don't have the emotional capacity to care. I cry myself to sleep thinking only of my Dad and how much I miss him while I listen to old voicemails from him over and over. I cry over the loss of a voicemail I once had of him singing me happy birthday. When he left it nearly eight years ago, I saved it as a recording, knowing I would play it for myself every year after he passed. But that phone died long before my Dad did, and I lost the recording. I mourn that loss, too.

NO HANDS AND A MARATHON RUNNER

TODAY I AM ASSIGNED TO a patient who can actually talk to me. His name is Tony, and he's been hospitalized for COVID for the past two months. He's on our unit while he waits for placement on the rehab floor. He's spent the past two months in the main ICU downstairs, but now that his status has been downgraded, they needed to move him to make room for someone sicker. He requires so much care that the doctors don't feel comfortable holding him on a regular MedSurg floor.

"Hi Tony!" I say as I enter his room. "I'm Laura, I'm going to be your nurse today. How are you feeling?"

"Helpless," he tells me with a sigh.

"Oh no. Why?"

"I can't use my hands!" he says with exasperation. "I'm useless without my hands. I ended up messing the bed last night because I had no way to get the nurse in here to put me on a bed pan before it happened."

"Oh no. I'm so sorry, Tony. I know the occupational therapist is coming by later today. Maybe she can help me come up with a way to make sure you can hit the call light. In the meantime, there's a camera right there. There's a nurse watching it twenty-four-seven. I'll let her know that if she sees you wiggling your feet and looking directly at it, to get me. But I'll also make sure to check on you at least every thirty minutes, O.K.?"

"I tried that last night. Whoever was watching the cameras either didn't see me or didn't care. I need my hands!"

"We'll do our best to find a way for you to be able to use the call light with your feet. I'll make it my top priority today."

Tony looks unconvinced but says O.K. so I can leave the room. My other patient, Sandra, is in a similar situation. She has a mental delay, and she's here for the second time this year. Her first visit a couple months ago was thanks to COVID, which led to her needing a tracheotomy and being admitted to a long-term care facility upon discharge. She's back due to sepsis from some sort of secondary infection she got at the long-term care facility. I've been told that last night's nurse struggled to get her off one microgram per kilogram per hour of Levophed, but the physicians really want it off. I turn it down to 0.5. Sometimes you have to titrate smaller doses than protocol says in order to get the patient completely off the vasopressor. I introduce myself the same way I did with Tony but am met with a blank stare and a grinding of her teeth that makes the hair on the back of my neck stand up. Sandra's mental delay includes a lack of speaking. I'll need to check on her as frequently as I do Tony to make sure she seems comfortable and looks clean, since she can't communicate her needs to me.

By the time I'm done charting the patients' assessments and gathering morning meds, a resident is harping me about Sandra's 0.5 micrograms of Levophed. "The attending wants it off," he tells me, an irritated look splayed all over his face. Point-five micrograms isn't even a dose. Just turn it off."

I sigh audibly. "I understand. I want it off, too. But the night nurse said she spent all night titrating her on and off of one microgram, which tells me just turning it off isn't going to work." I'm growing tired of having to explain how to practice medicine to physicians. It seems like after two years in the ICU, I have to explain something to an attending at least once a shift. And they're supposed to be the smartest person in the room. "Sometimes," I continue, "when a patient has required presser support as long as Sandra has, their body needs to be tricked into functioning without it. They require smaller titrations once you get the dose down to one to two micrograms in order to get it off and keep it off."

As if I haven't thoroughly explained anything, or even been talking at all for the last three minutes, the resident turns to me and says, "I'm going to turn it off when we go in there for rounds. We just want to see if she can keep her pressures up without it."

I roll my eyes. "O.K., but when it's back on at point-five micrograms in an hour, don't say I didn't tell you so." I instruct the person watching the monitors to keep a close eye on Sandra's blood pressure. I don't trust it to stay high enough.

Sure enough, as I'm in the middle of a new round of explanations with Tony's attending, the monitor tech tells me Sandra's pressures are dropping. "Hold that thought!" I tell the attending, who continues to talk over me, explaining the reasons it's unacceptable for Tony to be unable to hit the call light. As if I'm too stupid to understand that, or as if the warning that my other patient's blood pressure is dropping is of no concern since it isn't one of *his* patients.

This is another common frustration of mine. Nursing school is riddled with questions asking you to prioritize four things or situations that require your attention at the same time. The patient who can't breathe takes precedence over the patient whose blood pressure is tanking, which takes precedence over the confused older patient who's a fall risk and trying to get out of bed without assistance, which takes precedence over the patient asking for help getting to the restroom. What nursing school *doesn't* teach you is that, while these four things are happening, and while *you* know the order you need to attend to them and why, there will be people who care about only one of your patients and therefore will get angry when you don't place them as first priority on your list. The daughter of the patient needing to use the restroom will yell at you because her mom had to pee and you didn't get there in a timely manner to help. Never mind that someone else would've died if you had. The attending of the old man getting up will yell at you because he could've fallen, never mind that you would be running a code on one of your first two patients if you had helped the old man first.

Or, in this instance, never mind the fact that my other patient's blood pressure is tanking because the attending for my more stable patient is here right now, and he doesn't want to be delayed in speaking with me, because he has better places to be. Even though I clearly have somewhere better to be in this moment, too.

"Uh-huh. I'll be right back," I say again as I rip off my protective gear and push past him towards the door.

I don new protective gear, run into Sandra's room, turn the Levophed back on, strip the protective gear, sanitize my hands, put on new protective gear, and return to Tony's room, where the attending is telling him some restaurant called Spimoni's is too far away. "I'll get you some cannoli next time I'm in the pizza parlor down the street, though," he tells Tony. "Ah, there you are!" the attending says, acknowledging my return as if I had left to play a round of hopscotch and now it's time to move on to less frivolous matters. "So, as I was saying," he says, "there has to be a way to set this thing up so Tony can hit it with his feet. He *has* to be able to get ahold of you if he needs assistance."

"Yes, and as *I* was saying," I reply, putting as much emphasis on the word *I* as possible, "the night nurse tried that, and Tony ended up kicking it off the bed. This call light button is too small, and the medical tape is too flimsy to hold it in place, and Tony's feet are too weak to hope he can hit it every time unless we find a way to securely hold the call light still. I'm hoping OT will have either a better call light or a better solution. They should be by sometime later this morning."

Apparently, I'm talking to myself, because then the attending says, "Surely if we just tape it to the end of the bed he can hit it with his big toe."

I sigh. It's more of a huff, really. "You're welcome to try it. Please, be my guest."

The attending, of course, does not try it. Nor does he acknowledge that I've heard anything he's said or offered any solutions. "I'll make sure we get this straightened out," he says. "Tony, don't you worry! We won't allow any more accidents like last night while you're here."

"Yes, that was extremely unfortunate, and we're so sorry Tony. But," I say, looking at the attending, "the nurse who was caring for him was coding his other patient when that happened, and all their extra resources were in that code."

Again, priorities. And again, no one cares except the nurse, which is confirmed by the look on the attending's face.

In addition to assessing Tony and Sandra, charting those assessments, and giving them their morning meds, I have to feed Tony because his hands don't work. It's kind of awkward, because he can't talk while he's chewing. I've never fed someone who didn't have some sort of brain injury or stroke. His TV is on, but neither of us are really watching it. Between bites, Tony tells me that the attending always says he's going to bring a cannoli but never does.

Once he says he's done with breakfast, about half of what they brought for him, I spend about ten minutes making sure he's comfortable, just in time for occupational therapy to come in and say it's time for him to move to the chair. I'm behind on charting, and I need to check on Sandra, so I leave them be.

On my way to Sandra's room, I'm stopped by a nurse who introduces herself as Hailey. "You're taking care of Tony today?" she asks. "I took care of him all last week. How's he doing? He is such a sweet man."

"Yeah, he is! He's doing O.K., just sad about his hands. I guess he had a rough night last night, too. He had an accident while his nurse was coding her other patient. OT is working with him now. I'm hoping they can figure out a way to make the call light accessible for him."

"Awe, poor guy. I know he's super frustrated with his situation. Did he eat anything for you this morning? I had a hard time getting him to eat last week. He said he doesn't like the food here."

"I can't say I blame him. He ate about half his breakfast. I walked in on him telling his doctor he wants Spimoni's. Some sort of pizza place. I'm going to see if I can get it delivered."

"That's a great idea. Let me know how much it is, and I'll pitch in for half."

"That's super sweet of you. You don't have to do that," I tell her, pleasantly surprised at her generosity.

"Oh, I want to! I can't stand that doctor. Every day he jokes that he's going to bring poor Tony a cannoli, but I can tell Tony thinks he's serious. You shouldn't mess with patients like that. This isn't a joke to him."

I agree 100 percent.

I check in with Sandra. She's asleep, and her blood pressure looks stable. I turn the Levo down to 0.25 micrograms per hour. The next time I'm in there, I'm able to turn it off completely. I end up asking Hailey for help throughout my shift. She's assigned to someone else as a helper-nurse. For some reason I didn't get one today, but I figure there must be a reason, and I still feel too new to complain. We give Sandra a bath together after she has an accident. Then Hailey offers to feed Tony lunch so I can finally chart both my assessments.

"Are you sure?" I ask her.

"Yes, of course! You get your charting done, I'm happy to help. Plus, I'd love a chance to get to talk to Tony again." I don't know how I'd be surviving this job without the kindness of strangers.

I honestly don't remember a ton of details about the day. It's one of a handful of shifts where my patients aren't on the brink of death the entire time. My mind is so consumed with the difficult stories from COVID that I don't have much room left for the details of good days like these. But I will remember Tony. Tony will stick with me for many months after this day. So will Hailey and her kindness not only for me, but for her patient. I'm becoming so weary at this point in my contract that I'm losing the desire to check in on patients I had the week before. I'm losing the desire to help other nurses, because I constantly feel like I can't even help myself. Hailey hasn't lost that, though. She is shining with kindness and compassion for everyone around her.

In any spare time I have that shift, I google ways to get Spimoni's delivered, but there is only one in Brooklyn and it's five miles away, far enough that the restaurant won't deliver. I boil with irritation at Tony's physician. If I had a car, I would drive to Spimoni's for him.

Hailey and I settle for the pizza place a few blocks down from the hospital. Come dinner time I am too busy to leave the hospital, so Hailey offers to get the pizza. We want it to be a surprise for Tony, so we get one cheese and one pepperoni, figuring we can't go wrong with those choices. I give Hailey my credit card and insist that the pizza is on me, thanking her again for all her help today and her help now in actually getting the pizza. When she gets back, we take a picture together with the box, then we go in to surprise Tony together. He laughs and tells us we shouldn't have, but he looks happy. I let Hailey talk to him in between bites while I hold the pizza up for him. He makes fun of me for being a Midwesterner when, at first, I have to ask him how to hold it up. "Fold it!" he laughs. "Aye aye aye! Americans!"

"I guess I've been eating pizza wrong all my life, then," I tell him.

"No, you've been eating the wrong kind of pizza! If it's not too flimsy to eat un-folded, it's not Italian."

Hailey and I talk a bit with each other while Tony eats. He doesn't seem to mind. I think he likes our company, even when he isn't directly a part of the conversation. Hailey sees my watch through my protective gown and asks whether I'm a runner. "I am!" I tell her, excited because it usually takes one to spot one. "I used to be into triathlons, but with COVID and being in New York I've boiled it down to distance running."

"That's awesome!" Hailey exclaims. "I actually ran my first marathon in April. I've been trying to keep it up since I got out here."

"Oh my gosh, congratulations!" I tell her, giddy to have someone to share my passion with.

"We should totally go for a run together," Hailey squeals.

I tell her that sounds wonderful, but internally I panic a little, worrying that she'll be too fast to run with me.

"You girls be careful," Tony says. "I grew up in the Bronx, and I wouldn't be running out there by myself if I were you. Promise me you won't go running by yourselves. It's not safe." His paternal worrying is very sweet, and we both promise as we cross our fingers. When Tony has had enough pizza, Hailey and I make sure he's comfortable in his bed. He says all this commotion had been the best part of his day, but it has also made him ready for a nap. *Finally, a shift that can end on a good note.*

Hailey and I keep talking about running when we get into the hallway. I'm thankful I'm caught up on my patient care; this is one of the most exciting conversations I've had since I got out here.

Hailey echoes my thoughts by saying, "Oh my gosh, it's so nice to have someone who shares my passion for running. I'm such a geek about it. I could talk about it for days."

"I'm the exact same way," I tell her. We exchange books we've read and races we've run. She tells me that the marathon she registered for in April had been canceled, but she ran it solo anyway.

"That is beyond bad-ass," I told her. "I've only done a handful of halves, but I'm hoping to work up to a fifteen-mile run while I'm here in New York."

"I would love to run with you," Hailey says.

"Yes, me too! But I worry you'll be too fast for me. What's your mile pace?"

"Usually nine and a half to ten minutes, depending on how far I'm going."

O.K., I think. *It'll be a stretch, but I bet I can keep that up for at least four or five miles.*

"I've been planning on going out to this place called Roosevelt Island," she says. "Supposedly it's four miles around and there's a trail that wraps its perimeter. There's also an abandoned smallpox hospital and a lighthouse."

Four miles, perfect. "I'm in!" I tell her. Hailey has been much more adventurous with her runs than I have. She's also been taking the subway, something I have yet to do.

We get to talking about coaches. I used to have one but haven't bothered since my previous attempt at a 70.3 Ironman. "I love mine," Hailey tells me. "She's very good about being flexible with my nursing schedule. Each week is tailored around it."

"That's awesome. Do you have an Instagram?" Instagram has a pretty big running and triathlete community, and it's where I've connected with a lot of people in this sport thus far.

"I don't," she says. "I used to, but I found myself constantly comparing myself and my running accomplishments to other runners on there. I deleted it to keep myself from doing that."

"I can *totally* relate," I tell her. "I ended up injuring myself a long time ago trying to keep up with everyone else's speeds and distances."

"Exactly," she says. "Plus, I just really felt that at some point God was telling me I didn't need to share everything. Like I felt like He was asking me what my motives are. For example, did we buy Tony pizza today so we could tell

Instagram about it, or did we do that because we wanted to help out our patient? Sometimes it's O.K. to just keep things to yourself."

I feel like God reached down from Heaven and smacked me upside the head. All day I have been drafting captions in my head for the photo Hailey and I took with Tony's pizza box. I was going to post some bullshit about how "maybe I can't save everyone, but I could make this patient's day with a piece of pizza and that made my time here worthwhile."

I never share the photo. I've never even shared this particular story from my time in New York until now. But this conversation has stuck with me long after it happened. Hailey has that effect on people; her words tattoo themselves onto your heart.

After exchanging numbers and solidifying plans to go to Roosevelt Island for a run, Hailey leaves to help her nurse with end-of-shift things. I check on Sandra and do her final oral care and turn for the shift. I am almost done with my tasks when Sandra's heart rate shoots up from the seventies to the 150s. *Oh fuck. So much for the happy ending of my day.* I get a twelve-lead EKG, which confirms what I already know; Sandra's heart has gone into A-fib RVR, a dangerous cardiac rhythm. I page the resident, who orders the standard treatment of an amiodarone bolus and drip. I call pharmacy several times before finally getting the medication.

"I don't understand why this happened," the resident says. "She did this a week ago and we converted her out of it and onto oral amiodarone. She got that today, right?"

"Yeah, she did." I sigh. I don't understand it either.

"I honestly don't know whether this drip is going to help her or not. And we just got her off of the Levo."

I had to restart it when Sandra's heart rhythm changed. "Obviously her body can't handle being off of it, then," I say.

I stay late to hang the amiodarone drip that arrives after my nurse has gotten report from me. I would want the nurse to do that for me if the roles were reversed. When I finally get to the break room, I'm exhausted from all the last-minute chaos and very much looking forward to my share of the pizza I had gotten for Hailey and me. I find the box, with my name on it, empty on top of the trash can.

"Are you fucking kidding me?" I say to no one in particular. The night nurse sitting in the break room looks startled and asks, "What happened?"

"Someone ate my fucking pizza." I shake my head and storm off to head home. I don't have the emotional reserve to deal with shit like this.

Fuck it. I'll order DoorDash and have a beer in the shower.

ROOSEVELT ISLAND

ON SATURDAY, I SET OUT to meet Hailey at a subway stop for our trip to Roosevelt Island. She had already mapped out the route to get there when she invited me to join her. "Maps says we take this subway for about fifteen minutes, and then we walk five or six blocks over to an air tram that'll drop us off on the island."

"Oh my gosh. You can use Maps to get around on the subway? I had no idea. That would've made my vacation here last winter so much easier."

"Yeah, this is how I've gotten everywhere! Central Park, Rockaway Beach, a few places in Manhattan."

She tells me about her various adventures in New York during our subway ride. I tell her about running in Park Slope, which she also does regularly, and biking to the piers to run across the Brooklyn Bridge. "I've done that a couple times," Hailey tells me. "There's a subway nearby that will take you to and from Dumbo if you ever don't want to bike there." Dumbo is the name of the shopping district near the entrance to the Brooklyn Bridge.

When we get off the subway, we venture down a few blocks, climbing over a median in the street covered with tributes to the Black Lives Matter movement drawn on it in chalk and a few roses scattered at its base, and down along the East River.We pass under the Queensboro bridge, which is beautiful. The tram we have to ride to get to the island goes right along the bridge, so we get to see it up close and personal.

The tram is an adventure. It's the only way to get over to Roosevelt Island. We use our subway cards to get on. Once inside, it's standing room only with a handful of poles and railings to hold on to for balance. All four walls of the tram are made of glass, so we're able to see for miles in any direction. The site is overwhelming. The east side of Manhattan is on one side; Queens is on the other. The sea of skyscrapers is breathtaking.

Once we reach the island, we take some more photos before starting our run. There are huge red letters—"RI"— right when you get off the tram. Hailey and I take turns taking pictures of each other posing next to the letters. I take a few more pictures of the Queensboro Bridge from this angle.

"O.K.," Hailey says as she pulls up her watch's GPS. "Google said the island is just one big four-mile loop. Which direction do you want to start in?"

"Doesn't matter to me," I tell her. We decide to veer left— and soon learn this is the end of the island with the old smallpox hospital on it. We stop long enough to read the information cards posted on the gate protecting the building.

"Do you think there will be historical tributes to the COVID pandemic like this old hospital someday?" Hailey asks me.

"I don't know. It's kind of crazy to think they tried to isolate all of the smallpox patients in the city to this little island back then." According to the information card, this building was the first hospital in the country dedicated solely to treating Smallpox in 1856.

"If only COVID could be contained to an island this small," Hailey answers sadly.

We continue our run around the island. I am surprised to find it's easy to keep up with Hailey. Our conversations flow almost effortlessly. As we round the island, we get a beautiful view of the Manhattan skyline. Since we are on the outer part of the island the entire run, we spend four miles next to the Hudson River. I can hear waves lapping the lower part of the wall keeping us on shore, and the air smells like the sea. The sun is out, but it's not too hot.

At the other end of the island is a lighthouse. "I brought my GoPro in case we wanted to get some cool action shots," I say. "Would you want to take a couple with this lighthouse in the background?"

"Yes, let's do it!"

It's only half a mile from the lighthouse back to the tram. We take a picture of our GPS watches side-by-side, proudly displaying our shared miles, before hopping on the tram back to Manhattan. We stop for a smoothie on our way back to the subway, which we take to Brooklyn Bridge Park. At work last week we'd had several local nurses tell us about a pizza place in the park called Julianna's. Everyone who told us about this restaurant had a different version of the origin story, but everyone agreed it was some of the best pizza in Brooklyn.

Juliana's is located right next to another pizza place called Grimaldi's. The supposed origin story is that Mr. Grimaldi got caught up in mafia activity in the early thirties and lost the brand rights to his pizza shop. In 2012, Mr. Grimaldi opened a new pizza shop named after his mother, Juliana's, in the same building that housed the original Grimaldi's, and right next door to the new Grimaldi's. Supposedly, the new Grimaldi's has the name, but Juliana's has the original recipe.

Juliana's looked like a homey mom-and-pop shop on the inside, with lots of old pictures from the original Grimaldi's hanging on its walls. We take our pizza to go and eat it in Brooklyn Bridge Park, which overlooks the Manhattan skyline and Lady Liberty. Hailey and I take turns posing with our giant pizza before quickly devouring the entire thing. Our coworkers were right—this pizza is delicious.

The park is only a couple miles from Park Slope (where both of our Airbnb's are located), so we opt to walk home to allow us more time to talk. As we walk upon Barclays Center, we see a huge crowd of people gathered outside. Barclay's Center is topped with what looks like grass or turf, and several police are lined up on it, guns ready to aim at the crowd. It's truly a surreal image.

"They must be here for one of the Black Lives Matter protests," Hailey observes.

"It's kind of scary to see all those cops up there," I reply. "One wrong move and a lot of people could get hurt."

As I'm saying this, a small fight breaks out near the edge of the crowd, and we hurry away. As much as I would love to be a part of these demonstrations, a lot of them have become violent, and my desire for safety is beating out my desire to stand among the crowd. Jake and my mom have both begged me not to be involved in demonstrations. Hailey shares my same concerns. She has a husband waiting for her back in Texas, as well as two children to get home to at the end of her contract.

"It makes me kind of nervous just living on the ground floor of my apartment building," she tells me.

"Huh, I hadn't even thought of that. I guess I'm glad I'm on the second floor." I walk her back to her apartment, and then walk the remaining mile to my own. The streets are a little emptier than they usually are, and I feel a little less safe by myself than I've been feeling since I got to New York. I wonder how long all this will last.

THE SHITTIEST SHIFT

THE NEXT DAY, A NURSE named Leah is assigned as my helper nurse. I'm excited to be working with her, she has previous progressive care experience (progressive care units are a step-down from the ICU, and these nurses have more experience with ICU-level skills then MedSurg or Psych nurses do). We are told in huddle that this is the first shift where our unit will have only one charge nurse instead of two. The unit has two different sides with a long hallway in between. The charge nurses usually have more than enough work to keep them occupied with just one side. I have no idea how we're going to manage with just one charge nurse for both sides to share. Plus, I've never worked with this charge nurse before. The manager says her name is Karen. The manager also says this will be the first shift with reinstated managerial rounding to ensure that all patient IVs and foleys have the correct date labels on them. There's a unanimous groan among the nurses. We know joint commission efforts are important, but we also know they've been thrown to the wayside because we've been drowning just trying to keep patients alive, and we're not exactly out of the woods yet—on this unit or in the pandemic in general.

As Leah and I are waiting for Karen to tell us our patient assignment for the day, a new admission rolls past us into a room. Shortly afterwards, I learn she will be one of our patients. *Of course she will.* As Leah and I are waiting for report, we hear our other patient yelling, "Help me!" We hesitate—she's technically the responsibility of the night shift nurse until we've received report, and there's a chance we can't even help her due to our current ignorance of her condition. After a couple more "help me"'s with no night nurse in sight, we decide to don some protective gear and pop in to see what's wrong. The patient tells us she's done with the bed pan. I exchange an irritated look with Leah. There are a few tasks that are reasonable to leave for the oncoming nurse, but a code brown cleanup is not one of them. But it's our job, and she's our patient, so we do it—literally beginning our day with shit.

When we finally leave the room, we're bombarded by the night nurse. "Hey, are you guys taking care of Susan today? I've been looking everywhere for you to give you report." She sounds annoyed, and we meet her annoyance with our own.

"We were looking everywhere for you, too, but we couldn't find you, and Susan kept yelling for someone to get her off the bedpan. So, we did it," Leah tells her, matching her tone perfectly.

The night nurse's face softens. "Oh, my gosh, I completely forgot she was on that. Thank you guys so much. It's been a heck of a night. I just got her a little after midnight, and her blood pressure has been all over the place, not to mention I'm pretty sure she's confused. The physicians aren't entirely sure what's causing it, and my other patient is all the way at the other end of the hall. He's kept me super busy, too."

My face softens, too. I know how she feels—like she should be able to do it all, but she just can't. It's too much.

"She's just a COVID rule-out, but I honestly don't think she has it. She's not really having a lot of oxygen-related symptoms aside from occasional shortness of breath. It's mostly just a blood pressure issue. Hopefully they can figure out what's going on with her today."

By the time we're done getting report, the night nurse from our other room has emerged. "Hey," he says, sounding somewhat out of breath, "I apologize in advance, but as I'm sure you saw, this patient literally just got here, so I basically know nothing about her other than that they had to emergently intubate her and start multiple pressers about an hour ago after she coded on another floor. I think they said they did two rounds of CPR before they got a pulse back. She's COVID positive. The resident said she'd call the daughter and try to get a DNR."

Great. Two new patients, and neither night nurse knows exactly what's making them unstable right now. New patients are usually more work and stress than a patient who's been on the unit for a few shifts. It typically takes that long to fully figure out why a patient is unstable enough to require ICU-level care and then implement care measures to stabilize their condition. Although patients are still a lot of work once stabilized, their care becomes less frantic and more routine.

"Wait, if she's a known COVID-positive patient, should we be taking care of our other patient who's just a rule-out?" Leah asks me.

"Good point. I don't think we should." I want to address this with Karen before we officially assume care for both patients, but we don't have time.

"The new admit's blood pressure is dropping," we hear over the walkie talkies. We are met in the patient's room by the resident. I don't recognize her. It's the first week of June, so they're all different, and they're all new to the ICU.

"What pressers is she on?" the resident, Stephanie, asks me. I glance quickly at the IV pumps—I'm not sure what the answer is without looking. "Looks like Levophed and vasopressin."

"O.K., I'll put in an order for phenylephrine, too."

"O.K. thanks," I tell her as I start to titrate up to max on the Levo. "Do you think we could hang some fluids in the meantime just to hold her blood pressure over? Also, could you please ask whoever's at the monitors to call pharmacy and make sure I get the phenyl ASAP?"

"Yeah, sure. Give a bolus of LR, and if that doesn't fix her blood pressure before you get the phenyl, give another one."

Leah leaves the room to get the fluids. I don't even have to ask her. I'm so glad she has progressive care experience; I'm beginning to think I'm going to need all the help I can get to survive this shift.

I bump the Levo up slightly past max just to hold the patient's blood pressure steady until we can get the fluids started. Her name is Martha. She's a mess, and so is her room. Her body is laying in a sprawled-out position without any blankets on top, and there are no supplies in here. We don't even have extra IV pumps. I tell this to Leah as she starts to gown up to come back in with the fluids.

"O.K.," she says, handing me the LR. "You get this going and yell out to me everything you think we might need. I'll get it all."

"Thanks," I tell her, priming the bag and then getting it hooked up to Martha's IV. Slowly but surely, I'm able to come back down to the maximum amount of Levo allowed. Unfortunately, I'm not able to get it any lower.

Twenty minutes or so later we finally have the room stocked. "Let's get her better situated," Leah suggests.

"You read my mind."

As we roll Martha to get fresh sheets underneath her, we are met with another code brown. It's hardened and sticking to her back, indicating that she pooped a while ago and no one bothered to clean it up. I understand that saving her life trumps changing her sheets, but again, it's not an acceptable task to leave for the oncoming shift to deal with. And Leah and I have now had to deal with it *twice*. It's not fair to us, and it's certainly not fair to Martha. Who wants to lay in their shit for over an hour? As we're cleaning her up, I realize she doesn't have a foley catheter in yet. Or an OG tube. Two things that should always be placed when a patient is intubated. And the dressing on her central line is coming off, so I'll have to change it, or we risk losing the line. More tasks for us to do. Her blood pressure begins to drop.

"Quick, go grab a couple more bags of LR," I say, "and a pressure bag if you can. She's going to need that second bolus, and the faster we can get it in her, the more it will help." I call Stephanie in and radio for the monitor nurse to re-request my phenylephrine. I needed it about thirty minutes ago.

"Go ahead and give her two more boluses," Stephanie tells me. "I'll call pharmacy myself and make sure we get that phenyl."

"Thanks," I tell her. "Also, she doesn't have a foley or an OG tube. Can you put orders in for those and I'll put them in?"

"I'll throw in an order for a foley, but don't worry about an OG tube. I'll put one in later if we end up needing it, but I'm still trying to get ahold of the daughter, and I'm hoping we can de-escalate some of her care once I do."

"O.K., thanks." I have Leah grab catheter supplies and a new central line dressing after she's returned with more fluids.

Another hour or so later, and Martha has fresh sheets, a Foley catheter, a new central-line dressing, new IV dressings, and a clean room—and phenyl has been started. Throughout that hour, I'm told at least three times by the monitor nurse that I need to check on Susan's blood pressure, which is also dropping. I have flashbacks to my first shift in this hospital, when my patients were both intubated, on multiple pressers, and yo-yoing their blood pressures from super high to super low for most of the morning. The unfortunate differences between that shift and this one are that today my patients are in two different rooms, and they're not both COVID positive, so I have to be extra careful when running into my rule-out's room to not bring my other patient's COVID diagnosis with me. This is easier said than done since I don't always have the three to five minutes it takes to don and doff all my COVID PPE before one of my two patients needs a blood pressure medication titration again. I also have to talk to my rule-out patient every time I run in to fix her blood pressure, which makes each trip into her room take longer than it should. She's very upset because she wants to eat, and she doesn't understand that the doctors won't let her because they want to do a few diagnostic tests to try and figure out what's making her blood pressure drop. While I empathize with her and want to comfort her, I just don't have the time. Martha has been threatening to code again all morning.

One of the times I run in to address Susan's dropping blood pressure, I'm confronted with two residents I've never met before staring intently at the beeping IV pump. "Excuse me," I say as I practically push them both aside and frantically push buttons on the pump to get the Levo running again.

"We paused it just to see what would happen to her blood pressure, and then we couldn't figure out how to restart it."

Are you fucking kidding me? "What happens is her blood pressure drops," I scold. "Pretty quickly, I might add. Next time, ask me instead of testing it for yourself. And don't touch the IV pumps. In general, *never* touch a nurse's IV pumps. My other patient is extremely unstable. I don't have time to be running in here all the time. Thanks." I'm usually not so curt, but I don't have room for anything else right now. I have too much to do to be dealing with baby doctors who want to play with my patient's equipment.

Because Martha's blood pressure has yet to stabilize, I feel a sense of urgency and impatience every time I have to enter Susan's room. Even though she is very sick too, and her blood pressure hasn't fully stabilized either, she is less sick than Martha. Once again, I am having to fight with everyone—including doctors, patient family members, and the patients themselves—to actually prioritize my ability to perform nursing tasks and provide effective care for both of my patients. The resident caring for Susan is different from the resident caring for Martha, so neither of them cares about the blood pressure of my other patient because that patient isn't theirs. Susan doesn't care about the fact that I have a post-code COVID patient next door who is worse off than she is; she's agitated and confused and just wants to eat. It's overwhelming and exhausting to try to simultaneously prioritize patient care and please those around you. It's also overwhelming and exhausting to simultaneously have two patients with unstable blood pressures with unknown causes.

Both of my residents are placing new orders every twenty minutes. I've been so busy completing their never-ending orders and titrating blood pressure meds that come 11:30 a.m.,

I still haven't logged on to a computer or given either of my patients their morning meds. Leah by my side, I share this fact with the unit manager when she comes by to do her rounding, expecting her to realize that I need help, and to offer some, but she doesn't. "I'll just give you a couple more hours to get things situated before I look at the dates on your dressings and IV lines," she says. She dismisses my concern regarding having a known COVID-positive patient and a rule-out patient, stating that there's limited ICU staff today and her charge nurses did the best they could with assignments. When I mention the inappropriateness of one nurse having two patients who are new to the unit and this unstable, she agrees with me and ensures me that "we'll make sure to fix the assignment for night shift so these patients won't get paired together again."

"O.K. great, but how does that help us?" Leah says to me after the manager has walked away.

By 1:30 p.m., we *finally* have time to give our morning meds—which were due at 10 a.m. I have never given my meds late during this contract. Neither Leah nor I have sat down, logged into a computer, drank, eaten, or peed since we arrived to work. We've been too busy trying to keep both our patients' blood pressures from tanking. At 2 p.m., when we're done with meds, I tell Leah, who's chugging a bottle of water, that I think we're finally caught up.

"Great," she replies. "Then I'm going to go to lunch. I love you, but I need to go now. You can go as soon as I get back."

"Yeah, girl, of course. I'll be fine. Go get some lunch and take a break. You deserve it. Thank you so much for all your help this morning. I don't even want to think about what a day like today would be like without you by my side."

"I'm going to get a red bull from the pharmacy next door. Do you want me to grab you one?"

"Yes please! The biggest one you can find."

"You got it. See you in an hour!"

Shortly after Leah leaves for lunch, Susan's resident tells me the attending wants us to take her to CT at 2:30 p.m. "O.K. Do I need to go down with you?" I ask.

"Yeah. She's on multiple pressers, so I would feel more comfortable if you were there to manage them."

"O.K. I might have to find someone else to go with you. My other patient is extremely unstable, and I don't feel comfortable leaving her for that long. I don't feel super comfortable taking this patient to CT either, since her blood pressure has been so labile this morning."

"I know. I don't understand why we have to get the CT in order to treat her for a pulmonary embolism. We all know that's what she has. Try to get the vaso off before we go down. Then she'll only be on one presser, and it'll be less of a big deal."

"Welcome to my world," I tell him as I think, *Of course we have to verify the diagnosis we all know a CT will verify prior to treating it. Where the heck did you go to med school? You can't just give someone blood thinning medication to treat a clot and hope you're not wrong!* I shake my head, increase the Levo by ten micrograms, turn off the vaso, and then go to search for the charge nurse. I run into the manager first, so I let her know what's going on.

"O.K., no problem. Karen should be able to go down to CT with your patient. Just let her know."

When I find Karen a couple minutes later, she starts on a long tangent about how nurses here don't go to CT, that's the residents job. "Unless of course they're on pressers, and then we'll go down to manage the patient's IV drips."

"Yes, as I was saying," I reply, "my patient is on Levo at twenty to thirty, and vaso, so a nurse will need to go down with her, and I don't feel comfortable leaving the floor with my other patient on three pressers that need to be titrated every five minutes or so."

As if to prove my point, my walkie-talkie sounds: "Laura, Susan's blood pressure is tanking again."

"Don't worry, I'll go down with her," Karen yells after me as I run down the hallway to help my patient.

I'm hanging a fresh bag of Levo in Susan's room when a nurse named Steve pops his head in. "Hey," he says, "Karen told me I'm going to CT with your patient. Can you give me report?"

"Oh, O.K. I thought *she* was going down. Um, yeah, sure. She's a COVID rule-out, but they're pretty sure she has a PE, so they want to get a CT of her chest. Her blood pressure's been bouncing all over the place. I've yet to get the Levo below twenty micrograms. And the vaso was on, but the resident just asked me to turn it off. You might want to wait for another bag of vaso to get here from pharmacy before you go down, just in case you need it. The one she has is running low, and her pressure dropped just now when the Levo alarmed."

"Why would I need another vaso if hers isn't even on?"

"Well, I'm just saying, if you end up needing to turn it on you might not have enough—"

"I'll just go up on the Levo, then," he interrupts. "Why do they want to get a CT of her chest anyway if she's this unstable?"

"Well, *as I mentioned*, they're pretty sure she has a PE, and they'd like to treat it so they—"

I'm interrupted again, only this time it's by Karen barging into the room. "Laura, do you not hear them on the walkie?"

"Um, no I haven't heard anything. What—"

"Your other patient's blood pressure is crashing. You need to get in there! I told Steve to tell you."

"O.K., well, he didn't," I tell her, shooting him a glare as I push past her towards the doorway, tearing off my gown and gloves.

"Yes, I did. I sent him in here to take your patient to CT and to tell you that the other one needed your help."

"I'm not saying you didn't tell him to say that. *I'm saying* that he in fact did not share that information with me, and therefore, I had no idea," I say as I burst out of the room, into a new gown and gloves, and then into Martha's room.

I can hear both her IV pump and her monitor beeping. One of the IV pumps is flashing all sorts of different colored lights. I've never seen one alarming like this before. *Shit, her phenyl is off. No no no no no!* Her blood pressure is fifty over twenty, and her heart rate is trending downward, a sign that her body is preparing to code. I try to get the IV pump to turn off and back on, but it won't do anything. It just keeps screaming at me and blinking red and blue lights. I can't even get its door to open. I'm going to have to reprime the phenyl and program it in an entirely different pump, and I don't have any spares in the room. I don't know if I can accomplish that before Martha's heart rate flatlines.

Steve comes in behind me and tries take over. "Push epi. You need to push epi!"

No, I need to get this phenyl running again. "You do it," I tell him, too exasperated to explain what I'm doing and why it's more important than anything else right now. I realize he isn't wearing a gown or goggles. "She's positive!" I tell him. He ignores me and keeps telling me to push epi. The constant beeping of the malfunctioning IV pump, coupled with the constant warning beeps of the monitor telling me my patient's blood pressure is dropping with her heart rate, and now Steve barking orders, are causing sensory overload. It's like I've forgotten both what words are and how to use them.

I look up at the monitor. The epi Steve pushed didn't do anything, and I'm still priming the phenyl. Fuck. "Push Levo!" I scream at Steve over the beeping.

"No, push another epi!"

"No. Push LEVO!"

"I can't reach it," he tells me.

I frantically try to draw some up out of the IV line so I can push it, but my fingers are fumbling. I'm trying to move twice as fast as normal and my heart is pounding out of my chest, but it's all just causing my fingers to fumble more. Steve takes the syringe out of my hand and goes to push it, but it's too late. Martha is coding. Steve starts compressions and I frantically throw a sheet over her head to protect us from the COVID particles being pushed out of her mouth or ventilator tube.

"She's positive!" I yell at him again as I hit the code button and try to get the phenyl hooked back up to her central line.

"It doesn't matter," he tells me between compressions.

There is suddenly a flock of residents in my room, and they're all saying different things. None of them are wearing gowns or goggles. "She's positive! She's positive! You need a gown!" I try to tell them, but no one seems to hear me or care about what I'm saying.

The resident that gave me the orders for the boluses this morning, Stephanie, is asking me what happened, and I'm still struggling to find words. "Can I help you?" she asks me, seeing me struggling to get the IV lines untangled and get the phenyl reattached.

"I got it," I snap at her. I didn't mean to—I'm just so incredibly frazzled right now. *Why did this have to happen while Leah is at lunch?* Stephanie backs off. Steve is yelling at me to record and I'm frantically trying to find something to write on. I grab a gauze package and write on the back of it. Other residents are thinking out loud about what meds to give other than epi.

Amidst all of this chaos, Karen opens the door and yells in, "Laura, they're ready to take your patient to CT. Why don't you go down with her and Steve can stay here and run the code."

Are you fucking kidding me? This is my *patient. She is actively coding* right now. *I'm not going anywhere.* "I don't really feel comfortable with that," I practically scream at her.

"O.K., I'll go down with her then."

"That would be helpful," I bark at her as I try to discern whether Steve is yelling at me that he gave bicarb or that he gave *another* bicarb, and whether or not I even wrote the first one down, if there was in fact a first one.

"O.K., guys, let's call it," a doctor I don't recognize says. "This is her second code today, she's in her seventies, she's COVID positive. She's not going to make it."

Stephanie stops giving compressions. "Time of death, three fif—"

"Hey, wait," Steve says. "Look at her ART line on the monitor. There's a waveform. That means there has to be a pulse."

Steve, Stephanie, the doctor who had called the code, and I each grab a different pulse site.

"Yep," the doctor confirms, "that's a pulse. All right, everybody, she's back." Then, to me: "Don't increase her pressers anymore. If she codes again, she's not going to make it."

"I couldn't if I wanted to. They're all maxed out," I tell him.

"O.K., then just know we are not going to add any more." Then he tells Stephanie to try to get ahold of Martha's daughter again.

"Last time I spoke to her she was on her way up here. She wanted to see her mom and speak with us in person."

"Very good. Get this room cleaned up, then," he says to me.

Right. Thanks so much for offering to help.

Stephanie must notice the overwhelm and frazzle I'm feeling, because she walks over to me, puts both hands on my shoulders, and says, "Laura. It's O.K. You're doing a great job. Take a breath."

I take a deep breath with her, nodding my head. I still can't find words.

"Nothing we do for this woman is going to save her life, O.K.? You know that. I know that. Everyone in this room knows that. I'm going to do my best to explain it to her daughter and make her comfort care, O.K.? Don't worry about it."

"I know. I just . . ."

"I know. But it's O.K. I'll be back soon, hopefully with the daughter, O.K.? Just breathe."

I nod. I'm trying.

Everyone leaves. I look around the room; it's a mess. There are medication wrappers and empty syringes everywhere, and Martha is once again in a disheveled position, her arms flailed out randomly in the bed, her sheets bunched up, her head cocked at an awkward angle.

"Hey." It's my friend Patrick. "Are you O.K.?" he asks. "I popped in during the code, but it looked like there were too many people in here, so I didn't want to add to the chaos."

"Good call," I tell him.

"Can I do anything for you?"

"I just have to clean this room before her daughter gets here. She's on her way."

"Oh," he says, smiling and taking a looking around, "is that *all* you have to do?" He starts laughing.

I do too, and before I know it, I'm doubled over in hysteria. I can't stop. Patrick laughs with me for a minute, but then I can tell by his half-hearted single laughs that he thinks I should've stopped by now. I'm laughing so hard I can't breathe, which is only compounded by the fact that I have an N95 on. I get to a point where noise is hardly coming out of my mouth anymore, but I'm still doubled over cracking up.

"I'm just waiting for the laugh that turns into a sob," Patrick says, laughing nervously.

I get ahold of myself. "Oh man," I tell him. "I was waiting for that, too. I guess I'm good."

"I'd say you're losing it, actually. Have you eaten anything today?"

"No. Leah's at lunch now. I was going to go when she got back. I'll try to, anyways, but I have to stay in case the daughter shows up."

"O.K. Well let's take care of this mess."

When we're done about a half hour later, I thank Patrick profusely and tell him we can just keep the code cart in the room. We may need it again. Martha is still a full code. When we emerge from the room, I see Leah walking down the hallway, two giant Red Bull cans in her hands. "Oh my gosh, Leah!" I cry as I run over and hug her.

"Oh no. What happened?" she asks me.

"She coded, Leah. Ten minutes after you left, she fucking coded."

"NO SHE DID NOT! Are you serious?"

"Dead serious." In hindsight, my word choice is unfortunate.

"Oh no. Are you O.K.? Is she?"

"Yeah. We got ROSC. They don't want us to add anymore pressers, but her blood pressure is still pretty low. Her daughter is on her way."

"O.K., well that's good."

"Yeah."

Just as I say that we hear over Leah's walkie "Laura, her pressure is dropping again." Turns out my walkie is dead, and that's why I didn't hear them the last time they called me about Martha.

Shit.

Leah and I throw on new gowns and gloves and run in there together. Her pressers are all still maxed, and both her heart rate and blood pressure are dropping again. "Hit the code button," I tell Leah as I throw a sheet back over Martha's head and start compressions again. She does, and a few residents come running.

"Don't give any meds!" one tells us. "Just keep doing compressions. The daughter is here. We're going to bring her in."

"Is now really the best time?" I say between compressions.

"I think it's the only way she's going to let her go," he tells me.

Leah and I exchange looks of uncertainty. We continue to switch off on compressions every two minutes. Unlike a normal code, no one is bagging the patient. With COVID, bagging aerosolizes the virus more, and the danger that poses for healthcare providers far outweighs the minimal benefit it holds for the patient. Now that we've been instructed not to give code medications, compressions are the only thing that we can do. We both know that compressions alone are not going to bring Martha back. We also know that, even with bagging and code medications, Martha's time has run out; this is her third code blue today. We can't keep restarting her heart. But this makes very little sense to her daughter, who is still and wordless when she enters the room.

"They're doing chest compressions in order to circulate her blood right now," one of the residents explains. "If they were to stop, her heart wouldn't be able to beat on its own. This is the third time today we've had to do this." Stephanie explains.

The daughter just stares at her.

"These medications infusing through her IV were keeping her blood pressure up. They're still running now, but they're not enough to keep her heart beating anymore. The ventilator is breathing for her, and it's very likely that even if her heart were to restart on its own, we wouldn't be able to get her lungs to breath on their own. We've done everything we can to try to keep her alive."

The daughter starts shaking her head. It's almost in slow motion at first, and then suddenly, it becomes frantic. "STOP IT" she screams, shooing me and Leah away from her mom with her hands. "Leave her alone. Let her be. Let. Her. BE!"

Stephanie tells us we can cease compressions. Leah looks at me, uncertain. I nod my head and step away from the bed. The daughter moves to hold the hand of her mother's dead body. I shut off all the IV pumps and the monitor, which is now showing a flatline. The daughter is crying and screaming

"Why?" close to her mom's face without a mask on. I want to tell her it's unsafe, but I know she doesn't care, or she wouldn't be doing it. Besides, it's really the residents' job to say something.

The residents start to leave the room, so I do, too. I storm through the double doors to the other side of the psych-turned-ICU unit. I keep marching until I reach the rooms in the far back corner, which I know aren't being used and have padded walls. I enter one, shut the door, rip off my mask, and just start punching and kicking at one of the walls. "What the fuck?" I scream as I continue to beat on the padding. "What. The actual. FUCK?" I don't even notice the tears streaming down my face. I can't see. I can't think. I can't breathe. I've never had an outburst like this before.

In my head, that daughter is me. The patient I coded is my Dad. The residents standing around helplessly don't know how to save him as I stand by helplessly and watch. No one knows how to comfort me in my shock and grief. No one can. I am angry and sad and confused, and I already miss him so much more than I knew a human could miss another.

I catch my breath. I clean my face. I put on my mask. I go back to Martha's room.

"Hey," Leah whispers at me when I walk back in. "You or a doctor needs to talk to her. You and the residents just left, and all of a sudden, she had all these questions I can't answer. She's pissed, and I don't know what to say."

"I'm sorry," I whisper back. "I'll talk to her. Will you go ask whether one of the physicians will come in here, too?" I feel guilty for leaving Leah in there alone, but I'm equally angry that a resident didn't stay in the room. It's not within a nurse's scope of practice to discuss or disclose information related to the death of a patient. That falls to the physicians, and it's amazing how many of them can't seem to remember that.

"Can I get you anything?" I ask as I approach my patient's daughter.

"I'd say my mother, but you were apparently incapable of doing that," she says. My heart drops to the pit of my stomach. I can feel my eyes well up again, but I know my tears aren't welcome here. She will have no room or sympathy for grief coming from anyone other than herself.

"I'm so very sorry for your loss. We did everything we could. Can I get you a water or some tissues?"

"No. What you can get me is an answer for why this happened. She was fine. She was supposed to be going home today. Now she's dead, and I just can't understand that."

"I'm so sorry, ma'am. I can't imagine how frustrating and difficult this situation must be. I've only been with her since this morning, at which point her heart had already stopped once, so I'm unaware of the state she was in prior to my assuming her care."

"Well, I'm telling you she was fine, and now she's dead, and I would like somebody to explain that to me."

"Of course. Let me go get one of the physicians. They'll have a better picture of what all happened. Again, I am truly sorry for your loss."

She nods but says nothing more.

I storm into the physicians' room and bark at the several residents who were present for Martha's code that one of them needs to talk to the daughter. I ask them to escort her to another area of the unit so we can begin postmortem care on her mom's body.

Once the daughter and resident are out of sight, Leah and I gown up and began cleaning Martha and her room. As Leah rolls her onto a body bag, I can no longer hold back the tears that have been threatening to leave my eyes.

"I'm O.K." I tell Leah as we kept working. "I just need to be sad for a minute. I need it to be O.K. that I'm not O.K. all the time. Everyone always wants to make things better right away, but sometimes they're just not going to be. Sometimes I just need to be sad for one goddamned minute because something fucking sad just happened." I sniff. "But I'm O.K."

"I know you are," she says. "It's O.K."

"I'm just really sad because yesterday was my birthday and I didn't realize how much it would affect me, but I just really miss my Dad right now. It was my first birthday without him. I miss him so much. Every patient I loose feels like him, and every family member that dies feels like an extension of myself. I just miss him so, so much."

"I know you do," Leah said.

I'm beyond thankful for the space she's allowing me in this moment. Sometimes, I feel suffocated by my grief. As if I can't let myself and my feelings be the way they are because other people can't handle them, or because it feels inappropriate to express them. But Leah can handle it right now. I'm sure she feels some emotions of her own, too. Neither of us has ever coded a patient in front of their daughter before. Someone typically escorts family out of the room when a code happens, because it's a violent process and very difficult to witness.

Once we've finished caring for Martha's body and cleaning the room, Leah suggests I go to lunch. It's 5:30 p.m. I don't even know if Susan is back from CT or not, but Leah reassures me she'll figure it out and take care of Susan while I'm gone.

"Might as well call it dinner at this point," I tell her.

I grab the Red Bull she'd gotten me and a water bottle and head outside. I need to be anywhere but here. I do my best to avoid the gaze of others on my way out. I still need space to just feel sad. I walk down the street to my apartment, where I find my birthday present from Jake in the mail. AirPods—the only suggestion I'd given him other than a heartfelt letter, which does not accompany the AirPods in my mailbox. I'm happy to have something from him anyways, and too exhausted to feel any of the anger I felt towards him last night. I deposit the AirPods and my Red Bull in my apartment, grab my headphones, and head back outside. I don't know where I'm going, I just want to breathe in fresh air. I feel like I haven't been able to catch my breath since Martha lost hers.

I finally stop walking when I come upon a concrete ledge under some shade. I sit down, put my headphones in, take a sip of my water, and called Jake. "Hey," I say, "I know you're probably working, but can you talk? I just need you for a minute."

"Sure, babe. I'm actually driving home. What's up?"

Thank God. I just need to feel love from someone. I need to hear the voice of someone who loves me to replace the voice of the woman who holds me partially responsible for the death of her mother. "My patient died." I immediately start crying.

"Oh no. I'm sorry, baby."

"It's O.K.," I squeak. "I just need to be sad for a minute. I just need to talk to somebody who understands why I'm sad. I miss my Dad. He didn't call to tell me happy birthday yesterday because he can't, and that sucks, and I just really, really miss him."

"I know you do. I'm so sorry."

"I've never coded anyone in front of their daughter before. She was so upset. It was horrible. I kept thinking 'What if that was me?' That could've been me. This could've been my Dad."

"I know, but it wasn't. You got to be with him. The rest of his family got to be with him. This isn't him."

"I know. I just miss him so, so much."

Jake sits with me on the phone while I cry some more.

When I finally get a grip, I asked him whether it would be O.K. if I don't call again later this evening. "I have to go to work tomorrow, too, and at this point I'm not sure how I'm going to do that."

"Sure, babe. Feel better. I hope tomorrow goes O.K."

"Thanks. Me too."

I hang up the phone and dial my mom's number.

"Hi sweetheart!" Her typical greeting.

"Hey," I say, "how are you?"

"Oh, not too bad. How are you? Did you work today?"

"Yeah, I'm on my lunch break right now."

"Lunch? It's 6 p.m. your time!"

"I know. My patient died."

"Oh, honey, I'm so sorry."

"Thanks. I'm O.K. There wasn't anything else we could've done. I just miss Dad." With this sentence comes more water works.

My mom begins to cry as well. "I miss him, too," she chokes.

"I'm sorry," I say. "I didn't mean to upset you. I just needed to talk to somebody who gets it, you know? Everyone sees that I'm upset, and they want to fix it and ask if I'm O.K. Well, no, I'm not fucking O.K. My patient died, my Dad died, everyone's dying. It sucks. I need for it to be O.K. that I'm not

O.K.. I just need to be able to be not O.K. sometimes, you know?"

"I know," she says.

Someone walking past me looks in my direction, waves sheepishly, and says, "Thank you." To this day it is the most profound thank-you I have ever received as a nurse. That lady clearly knew I was a medical professional since I was sitting on a curb in scrubs, and anyone around me could tell that I was crying. I feel deeply touched that she chose to acknowledge my situation. Most people would've avoided eye contact.

"I woke up feeling kind of sad," I tell my mom, "because when I got home last night I realized how much I miss having Dad around on my birthday. I didn't realize it was going to affect me this much, but it did. He always used to call and sing me 'Happy Birthday.'"

"That's right, he did. I didn't even think about that. I'm so sorry. I could've called and sang 'Happy Birthday.'"

"It's O.K., Mom. I would still be missing him even if you had."

"Well, of course. You two used to always do something special together on your birthday since it was so close to his. Of course you miss him more now than you did on his birthday. Your birthday is when you two always celebrated each other."

"Yeah. I don't think I've missed him this much since he died."

"I'm so sorry honey. He loved you so much."

"I know he did. Thanks, Mom."

"Do you have to work tomorrow?"

"Unfortunately."

"Are you sure you can handle it?"

"Do I really have a choice?"

"It's ultimately up to you. You could always say you're not feeling well. Don't push yourself, O.K., kiddo?"

"O.K. I love you. I've gotta go. My break is almost over."

"O.K. I love you, too."

I walk back into work puffy eyed and red faced.

"Hey, did lunch help?" Leah asks as I walk up to her.

I shrug.

"Are you here tomorrow?" asks the monitor nurse.

"Yeah."

"Jesus. No one would blame you if you called in. You get shit on a lot. It's got to be getting to you. I feel like one of your patient's dies every time I work with you."

"Yeah, it's starting to feel like that to me, too."

"You should really call in," Leah says. "No one would blame you at all. Your mental health is just as important as your physical health. You're clearly not O.K., Laura."

I nod slowly. "I just miss my Dad so much," I choke out, tears stinging my eyes again.

"Please just call in," Leah says. "You deserve it. Take a day for you. Dedicate it to your Dad."

"O.K. You're right." I'm nervous as I call in. I don't have a reason in mind, but they don't ask for one. The woman in the scheduling-office just tells me to "Feel better soon" before hanging up. That settles that.

The rest of the shift is a blur. I get through it a lot easier than I expected to knowing I don't have to come back the next day. Every cell in my body feels heavy. So many people are dying. So many people are hurting from the loss of their loved ones. It's all I can think about. I go home, put on *Mean Girls*—a movie I've seen countless times before, and is both lighthearted and silly, the exact opposite of today—and mindlessly drink whiskey until I drift off to sleep. I don't call Jake to tell him I've called in. I'm worried it will upset him, since the whole reason I'm here in New York is to work. But I just can't do it. I can't do anything, right now. The grief I feel is all-consuming.

I wake the next morning in tears. Ellie, my dead puppy, is the first thing I think of. I don't know why I'm grieving her now instead of my dad, but I've learned that grief never moves in a straight or sensible line. I start scrolling through pictures and videos of her, letting the tears fall as I do. I did the same thing one morning with pictures and videos of my Dad. It's depressing and not fun, but for some reason it helps. After that, I put a movie on: *King of Statin Island*. It just came out, and Jake must have rented it last night because it's available on our Apple account. Eventually, I decide I need to get outside and get some air. I grab a book, a beer, and a blanket and head to the park. Shortly upon entering, I passed a scraggly-looking homeless man sitting on a bench digging through a barely filled trash bag. I burst into tears again. *What the fuck is wrong with the world that this poor man has to dig through a nearly empty trash sack in the middle of a park in New York to find food? Why don't I have anything to offer him? Why is everyone O.K. just walking past him as if he doesn't exist? The world is going to crap.*

I try to get a grip. I chug the beer I brought. I put in my new AirPods. I don't even pretend to try to read my book. I know I don't have the concentration in me. I stare up at the trees, listening to the lyrics of my music, and allowing time to pass me by. At some point I open my eyes. I see a man playing frisbee with his dog. I burst into tears again. People probably think I'm crazy, but I don't have the energy to care. Then it starts to rain. I sit in it for a minute, trying to clear my head. I finally pack up to leave when I realize my book is getting wet. Once I'm back at my Airbnb I open the whiskey again.

CONVERSATIONS AT CONEY

THE NEXT MORNING IS KINDER. Anna and I have plans to go to the beach. She lives in New York and wants to show me Coney Island. "Even though it's not its usual self right now," she told me with a smile.

She greets me at my apartment around noon carrying a vegan matcha birthday cake with candles and a small gift.

"Anna, you didn't have to do this," I say. "Thank you so much! This is truly the sweetest thing anyone has done for me for this birthday." She has gotten me a card in my favorite color. "Orange! You remembered!"

The cake is vegan because she knows that I don't eat dairy (it doesn't agree with my stomach), and the gift is a small Russian Matryoshka doll (Anna is originally from Siberia). "So you'll always have something to remember me by," she says. To this day, it sits on my vanity, where I can see it every morning.

We walk to the subway stop, chatting the whole way. I tell her about the horrible shift I had two days ago, and about how I felt really sad on my birthday because it was the first without my Dad.

She validates everything I say and tells me I'm very insightful for my age. No one has ever told me that before. It's nice to hear.

Just as I'm thinking that Anna feels like the big sister I've always wanted, she says, "You feel like a little sister to me. I love you." It's the most wonderful thing I've heard since the day I landed in New York.

The rest of the day continues like that: talking about our childhoods, our parents, our nursing career, our relationships, our lives before and after the start of COVID. I feel like I can tell her anything. I hope she feels the same. I think she does.

The beach is literally a breath of fresh air. It's the first place I've removed my mask in public since the start of the mandate. It's definitely the first time I've removed it in public in New York. I've even done all of my runs prior to this day with a Buff on, just in case. My feet in the sand, saltwater scents filling my nose, the breeze blowing my hair—it's perfect. We talk for hours, and for the first time in months, I'm not focused on COVID, not stressed, not hiding from the world around me. I just am. I think that day trip saves my life. The shore grounds me and reminds me that I am merely a grain of sand in the ocean of the world, washing away with the waves like all the patients who have been swept away before me. And yet, at the same time, we're all a part of something important. Something tangible. Something great. Something bigger than ourselves, or what we can see.

Over the course of my stay in New York, I will come back to Coney Island three more times. On the days that I need to feel both centered and free, the beach helps ground me. Every time, it reminds me that there are much bigger things happening in the world than all the things that seemed to be happening to me.

At the end of our day trip to Coney, Anna promises to have her husband, Martin, take us to Rockaway beach the next week. "You either have to take the ferry or drive in order to get there, but Martin loves Rockaway so I'm sure he'd be happy to drive us."

The night before we're supposed to go to Rockaway, my conversation with Jake somehow turns into a huge fight.

"Laura, you promised you would quarantine for two weeks when you got home from your contract. That's a big part of the reason I was O.K. with you going!"

"I know, Jake, but that was before testing was so readily available. My hospital now allows staff to get free COVID- and COVID-antibody testing. I can get tested the day before I fly out and guarantee that I'm not bringing COVID home with me."

"What if you get it on the plane?"

"Jake. I'm going to be wearing the exact same N95 mask that I've been wearing at work the past thirteen weeks on the plane ride home. If I haven't caught it by the end of my contract from being *directly exposed* to *known COVID positive patients*, I *highly* doubt I'm going to pick it up on the plane."

"But you just can't know for sure. And you promised, babe. I feel like this is you not taking my fears seriously again. You disregarded my concerns for my safety when you first started working with COVID patients here, and now you're doing it again. Just so you can live more comfortably. And I feel like you're not as careful as I am!"

"Are you fucking kidding me? How am I not as careful as you? If anything, you go out way more often than I do. You said you've been hitting up outdoor bars with our friends again. You think I'm doing that here? I wear a mask on the subway, I wear a buff when I run, my N95 is glued to my face for thirteen hours straight every time I work a shift. By the time I get home I will have been gone for *thirteen weeks*. I'm miserable. I fucking miss you. I miss Simba. I miss Rieger. I miss sleeping in my own bed. I would not be suggesting this if I didn't feel confident that you will be safe. I will get tested every day the week before I come home if that will make you feel more comfortable! How can you not want to see your own goddamn wife after thirteen weeks apart?"

I'm furious. How could he say that I—a COVID ICU nurse—am not as careful he is? I have other friends working contracts at my hospital who are married, and their husbands plan weekend trips up to see them and send care packages, letters, etc. Jake refuses to visit for fear of his own safety—which I knew and accepted as the case going in—and hasn't sent me anything other than the AirPods I got for my birthday. The first two weeks I was here, I sent him multiple letters. I've stopped doing it because he didn't really seem to appreciate them, and he hasn't reciprocated my efforts. And now, even though I can guarantee a COVID-negative status, he's *still* not going to pick me up from the airport? I can't bare the thought of spending two weeks alone in a hotel within walking distance of my home, my husband, and my pets (a cat, Simba, and a dog, Rieger) after being away for thirteen weeks. I long for home and my husband more than my lungs long for air, and it hurts me deeply that he doesn't seem to feel the same way.

"Fuck you!" I scream into the phone through my tears, hanging up before I can hear his response. I grab my bottle of whiskey and head to the bathroom. I kneel on the side of the tub. I'm dry heaving in between sobs that are so violent I can't breathe. My efforts to slow my breathing only seem to make it worse.

The good news is that, unlike my previous two panic attacks, I seem to be aware that this one is happening. I know I can't pull myself out of it, so I dial my friend Emily. Both a nurse and a mom, Emily has the exact tone of understanding and support that I know I need right now. I'm still sobbing loudly, taking the occasional swig of whiskey from the bottle between gasps of air, as I sit on the floor of my bathroom and relay the fight I had with Jake to her, and how exhausted and lonely and sad I am in general because everyone's dying and it's fucking depressing and I still have to do this for six more weeks.

Emily later told me that she could only understand about half of what I was saying, but that was enough to give her a general idea of how to console me. Somewhere in the middle of our conversation, I remember that I was prescribed Xanax for situations exactly like this one. I take one with a big swig of whiskey as I continue to cry in dismay on the bathroom floor.

I wake up in my bed, my eyes so swollen I have to ice them for a full ten minutes before I can get my contacts in. I don't remember how long I talked to Emily. I don't remember how much whiskey I drank, or when I went to bed. The whiskey bottle is half-empty on the floor of the bathroom next to the Xanax bottle. My phone says I talked to Emily for nearly an hour. It also contains a text message from Brad that I have zero memory of receiving or responding to, asking whether I'd want to grab a bagel with him this morning before his flight home to Kansas City (to which I responded yes at some point last night).

I don't really feel hungover. More like I'm coming out of a coma. Like I felt so many feelings last night that I don't have any left. When I'm done icing my eyelids, I quickly pack a bag for the beach and throw on some sunscreen and mascara. I'm throwing my hair into a braid when Brad calls. "Hey," he said, "I'm off work. I'll wait for you at the end of your street."

"O.K., I'll be right there."

We sit on a stoop at the end of my street with our bagels. He tells me how his last shift went, and what his plans are for once he gets back home. His contract was originally supposed to last as long as mine, but he's called it quits early. He says he's excited to be able to spend the Fourth of July with this family later this week.

"I feel like I should take a picture or something," he says, shrugging in the direction of our hospital. "This is kind of a moment."

I shrug. My moment feels very far out of reach. I just want to be done. I just want to be home. I just want to be *wanted* at home. I say none of these things to Brad.

When Anna pulls up, I hug Brad an envious goodbye and hop in the car, excited to be getting away for the day. We stop at a Starbucks down the street. While we're waiting for our drinks, a man comes in carrying a small dog and lacking a mask on his face.

"Sir," the poor Starbucks employee tells him, "you have to have a mask on. And you can't have your dog in here."

"I'm in a hurry," he replies. "I'm running late. I just need a coffee." After several minutes of rummaging through his bag while muttering to his dog, who is sitting quietly at his feet, he half-heartedly puts a bandana around his neck, as if simply possessing a mask-like item redeems him from actually having to cover his nose and mouth with it.

The beach is perfect. Rockaway is much more beach-like than Coney Island. It's much less crowded, the waves are huge, and there are surfers on them. A seagull attempts to eat breakfast from a cluster of mussels that have washed up on the sand. A ton of large seashells, unbroken, have washed up along the shore. As Anna and I walk and talk like we did at Coney, I collect a seashell for each of my close friends back home. A piece of my summer. A piece of this chapter of my life.

It's a warm, sunny morning, and Anna and I swim in the ocean together, periodically getting washed over by the large waves crashing onto the shore. She gets out almost as quickly as she gets in; the water is cold. But I float in the sea for a while, letting the waves move me as they wish, looking up at the sun and the clouds in the sky as the rest of the world disappears, letting my fears and worries and sadness wash away with the sea. It's the most blissful moment of my entire trip. All of time seems to melt away in the sun.

We're only able to stay for the morning. Eventually, a storm creeps up behind the beach, and once lightning is visible the lifeguards make us leave. But the half hour we spend lying between the waves and the thunder are almost as blissful as my moment in the ocean. They're my two favorite sounds in the whole world, and my two favorite things in nature to watch. Water above and below, washing the world clean.

FIFTEEN-MILE RUN

Prior to the outbreak of the COVID craziness, I was training for my first half Ironman. I was about five weeks out from the race when it got canceled due to COVID concerns. Shortly after, I started picking up extra shifts at the hospital and gave up training entirely. Other than doing compressions wearing a PAPR, I didn't really exercise in the month leading up to New York. Aside from a couple of very long walks to the Brooklyn Bridge, I didn't exercise in New York either before I started running again. It didn't seem safe at my original Downtown apartment. But at my Park Slope apartment, I was merely blocks away from Prospect Park.

Prospect Park is beautifully green and full of various walking and running trails made of various terrain. There is a large pond in the middle of the park and a waterfall along one of the park's inner trails. It's essentially the Central Park of Brooklyn. The first Sunday I had off after moving to Park Slope, I decided to walk to the park and go for a jog. I made it about two miles before Jake called. I spent our call walking around the park, exploring my various trail options.

The next day I decided to take a Citi Bike down to the Brooklyn piers. There was a bike dock right outside of my hospital, and two bike docks along piers one through six. The trip down there is slightly over two miles and there are bike paths to follow nearly the whole way down. I ran about two miles up and down the piers before settling on a pier bench in front of Lady Liberty and the Manhattan skyline. The view was truly a site to behold. I FaceTimed Jake so I could show him. I could've sat there for hours.

I returned to that view on many of my days off. Though I only made it two miles the first time, I quickly turned two into seven, and seven into ten. After my first ten mile run along the piers and across both the Brooklyn Bridge and the Manhattan Bridge, I decided I wanted to work my way up to fifteen miles. I had never run farther than a half marathon before, and although far from a half Ironman, it seemed like a challenge worth being proud of accomplishing. I never made myself run on days I didn't want to, but I found that on most days off I genuinely looked forward to my run. My thoughts and I could get lost for hours staring at the skylines and watching the waves of the Hudson Bay. I found several routes that pass by Lady Liberty. My favorite route by far starts along the Brooklyn piers and continues across the Brooklyn Bridge to the Manhattan piers and back through Brooklyn Bridge Park towards home.

The morning after my trip to Coney Island with Anna, I set out on this favorite route of mine. My heart felt heavy still from the loneliness of my birthday, the heaviness of the Black Lives Matter movement and all of the protests that were going on, and the sorrow of the loss of my patient a couple days ago, compounded by all of the other patients I had lost.

Once I crossed the Brooklyn Bridge into Manhattan, I turned right instead of my usual left. I had recently read online that the trail along the bay of Manhattan circled all the way around the island, totaling thirty-six miles. I never set out on an individual run with a true distance goal in mind. I ran as long as I was feeling good, and once I started to near seven or eight miles in Manhattan, I'd typically head back towards the bridge to make sure I reached the bike docks before I ran out of steam.

That day's run was feeling particularly therapeutic. I let my mind wade through the slew of emotions I was harboring. I wanted to cry and scream, but instead, I pushed harder. Around mile eight, I was thinking of the mom I had lost three short days ago. Of the sorrow and contempt her daughter had shown towards us and the situation. I told myself that I had to forgive myself. I repeated it over and over in my head as I ran faster and faster. *You have to forgive yourself for all the people you've lost, and all of the people you've yet to lose. You have to forgive yourself for losing Ellie. You have to forgive yourself for not realizing the racism that has been taught to you—and do the work to unlearn it. You have to forgive yourself for the current stresses you are feeling in your marriage. You are only human. You are only one person. Everything happening right now is bigger than you. You are doing the best you can. You have to forgive yourself for the fact that your best doesn't feel like enough lately. Forgive. Forgive. Forgive.*

As I ran to this mantra of self-forgiveness, I decided I wanted to run a half marathon today. I had completed a couple of twelve mile runs while in New York and told myself I'd do a couple of half marathons before officially attempting my fifteen-miler. *Today will be my first half marathon,* I thought. The majority of my run was along the Manhattan pier. I ended up going through China Town to get to the Manhattan Bridge. I stopped by a bodega to refill my water pack and grab a couple snacks, knowing that my gels alone would not be enough to make it a full half marathon in this heat. I also grabbed a small

Red Bull and sipped it throughout my mile across the Manhattan Bridge.

Miles eleven and twelve along the Brooklyn piers really hurt, but my banana and Red Bull must have kicked in somewhere between miles twelve and thirteen, because suddenly, my legs didn't hurt anymore. *Might as well keep going,* I decided. Instead of grabbing a Citi Bike to ride the remaining two miles back to my Airbnb, I kept running. I was feeling euphoric now. It was as if I had shed all the unfavorable feelings I was carrying back in Manhattan. I felt at least ten pounds lighter. Once I made it to thirteen and a half miles, I knew today was the day I'd run fifteen.

The last mile was nearly entirely uphill, and I started to hurt again. I decided to spend the last mile contemplating my own personal ignorance regarding white privilege and systemic racism. I reflected on ways I had been ignoring the problem, and ways I could take action in the future. I spent the final eight minutes running straight uphill as fast as I could with my mask on, reflecting on how it might feel to be strangled to death. To not be able to breathe because of another human being. To see light fade from the periphery of your vision but not see anyone around you offer you help. To be afraid of those who are supposed to protect you, in a country where "justice and liberty to all" is not actually inclusive of you and those who look like you. To know that so many in the world immediately judge you based on the color of your skin.

I can't imagine it. I can't even come close. But I do know that I owe the Black community my acknowledgement and support, and I alone am responsible for my own personal education and awareness regarding this movement. If it's not O.K. for people to suffocate from breathing tubes made necessary by a virus, then it is unacceptable for others to suffocate at the hands of a man, and it is absolutely intolerable that it happened to someone because of the color of their skin.

I hit fifteen miles at the Grand Army Plaza on the far end of Prospect Park, smack in the middle of a BLM demonstration. I take my mask down, catch my breath, and smile.

LIBERATION

THE FRIDAY OF MY ELEVENTH week in NYC, I wake ten minutes earlier than normal to make my final credit card payment. I did the math the week before, and throughout these eleven weeks—including today—I've paid off $23,466 in credit card debt. I followed Dave Ramsey's debt snowball method and paid them off smallest to largest: T. J. Maxx, Chase, CareCredit, Target, American Express, Amazon, Discover, Bank of America. Eight credit cards gone thanks to the fruits of my labors over eleven weeks and approximately 528 working hours. I make a cup of coffee, grab my Bank of America credit card and some scissors, and bask in the surreal feeling of being credit card-debt free.

I had credit card debt for seven years, since the day I turned eighteen. In high school, I heard Dave Ramsey's warning to not go into debt for anything, but I also heard the teacher of my finance class tell us that getting a credit card and always paying it off was the easiest way to accrue a credit score. I had also watched my parents use debt to make up for money they didn't have my entire childhood. My mom was the one who encouraged me to have a credit card once I started college. She said it could act as an emergency fund in case something were to happen to my car or I needed to front money for a college class or something. I'm pretty sure I used it the day after I got it to go shopping.

I did a decent job of staying out of debt my first year of college. Since I was undecided on a major, I used my A+ Program (a tutoring program my high school had, where we could earn two years of community college tuition in exchange for tutoring younger kids for free) money to attend the nearest community college in the evenings while I worked full time at a Starbucks during the day. I didn't use my credit card often, and I was always able to afford the monthly payment. I didn't have very good saving habits, although I'm not sure I really even made enough money to be saving it.

By the end of my first year of college, I was convinced I wanted to be a business major. I wanted more of a "college experience," so I applied for the University of Missouri-Kansas City's business program. I was accepted, and I began taking out loans to pay for school, which I attended on my two days off from my full-time job. After a semester of their business program, and a promotion at Starbucks that included more behind-the-scenes responsibilities, I decided business was not the route for me. I had made a friend in my math class who was pre-nursing and had heard her talking for the entire semester about the program and her reason for wanting to be a nurse. She seemed very passionate about it, and I wanted to feel that passion too. I also wanted to work closely with people, something I missed doing when I was given more business-focused responsibilities at Starbucks.

So, with two weeks left in the semester, I changed my major to pre-nursing, enrolled in all the prerequisites for the nursing program, and submitted my application. I got accepted, and, as is probably obvious, that was the major that managed to stick and turn into a career. While I wouldn't change that for the world, it was also the thing that rapidly increased my debt accumulation.

Not only did the nursing program cost more money, it cost more time, which made it seemingly impossible to work full time (although my best friend in the program managed to do it, and we ended up with the same new-grad job, so maybe I just lacked her tenacity). I quit my full-time job and moved downtown so that I could be closer to campus and my clinical sites. I managed to get a part-time job at an Aldi's down the street from my house, but the fifteen hours a week I was working felt difficult to manage. I was *finally* passionate about school, and I wanted to be all-in and acing my classes, not skating by on passing grades.

After my first semester of the program, I quit my part-time job. I managed to get a full-time summer job serving poolside drinks at a local country club. In hindsight, I should have saved all that money for the following semesters, but instead I bought an expensive triathlon bike, along with a nice bike trainer and grade-A bike kits. I had met a girl in my nursing program who did Ironmans, which I'd never heard of before but immediately became entranced with, and was eager to get into myself. I thought I needed gear like hers to be good at the sport, so I put rationale aside and spent money I didn't have on gear I didn't yet need. I do think the sport got me through the final two years of the nursing program—it was a difficult program and the exercise helped with my stress—but my part-time campus job was not enough, financially.

In addition to school loans, I began to take out more credit cards. I got a Discover card while working at Aldi's because it was the only credit card they accepted. Discover gave me a rather large credit limit, and the number excited me so much that I began applying for other cards, hoping to receive similar credit lines. I used them to pay for triathlon gear, groceries, gas, drinks, and more. My final year of nursing school, I maxed out the Discover card paying for physical therapy and chiropractor appointments after injuring my hip while training for a race. I didn't have health insurance, so I had to pay full price for each appointment, and I was required to go twice a week for nearly two months. I bought a couch I couldn't afford because I got tired of sitting on Jake's futon, and at some point in nursing school, my paid-for car died an irreparable death, and I ended up taking out a car loan as well.

By the time I graduated, I was drowning in debt. I now had five credit cards, a car payment, and several large student loans. I had thought it would be easy to pay off once I started my nursing career, but Jake and I made the stupid decision to upgrade our apartment to a downtown, two-bedroom, luxury unit. A decent amount of my increased income went towards paying my increased rent, and I had vastly underestimated the cost of the minimum payments on my student loans. With my first big-girl paycheck, I had to make minimum payments on five credit cards, four student loans, and my Prius. After the cost of rent, utilities, and groceries, I was pretty much the same level of broke that I had been while in Nursing School.

Fast-forward a year and Jake and I were paying for a wedding and a new puppy. When she got sick, I took out three additional credit cards in attempt to afford her vet bills. It got to the point that, some months, I didn't even make my minimum payments. My parents didn't have money to spare, and I was too embarrassed about the mess I had gotten myself into to admit this all to Jake. Besides, he paid for a lot of things while I was in nursing school, and I didn't think asking him to pay for more things was a very nice way to pay him back that favor now that I was out of school.

When COVID hit, there was talk that his law firm might go under, and the genuine panic that that gave me was enough to push me towards this NYC contract. After my first paycheck from the contract, I was up to date with all my minimum payments. And now, after eleven weeks of strenuous work, I am eight monthly payments and $23,466 lighter. Surreal is the only word I have for how it feels.

Each time I paid off a credit card, I cut it up into tiny pieces and closed the account. Now I do same thing with my final credit card, the Bank of America one, as I enjoy my morning coffee. When I get to work, I make a sign that says, "Credit Card Debt Free: $23,466" and have my coworker take a picture of me holding it up, my smile so big it's visible through my mask. I post it on my Instagram account, and three days later, Dave Ramsey himself reposts it on both Instagram and Facebook. There is no personal accomplishment I have ever been more proud of, and that surreal feeling—plus the financial freedom that accompanies a lack of monthly payments—makes all the difficulties of this contract worth it.

TO DIE OR NOT TO DIE?
THAT IS THE QUESTION.

IT'S PAST 8 A.M. AND I still haven't received report on my patient. His night nurse has been running around like a madwoman. "I'm so sorry," she says in a huff as she finally sits down next to me. "My other patient has been a shit-show since he got back from surgery at 3 a.m. He's all messed up from the anesthesia. He keeps saying I'm the devil and won't let me touch him, but he has a GI bleed, so he needs to be frequently cleaned up, not to mention his vitals have been less stable since he came back. And now they're talking about possibly starting CVVHD, and they're going to give him to a PCU nurse today. I swear I am this close"—here she holds up her thumb and forefinger pinched together near her face— "to quitting this contract. Giving a patient this sick to a PCU nurse is just negligible care."

"Oh, that's weird. Is your other patient on CVVHD?" I ask.

"No, so I can't understand why they aren't giving that patient to her and this one to you."

I sigh and say that I agree. "Why don't we ask them?" Then, turning to the PCU nurse down the hall, I say, "Hey

Diane, do you want to trade patients? The one I was supposed to get isn't on CVVHD."

"Yeah, that would be great. I'll double check with Kelly that that's O.K., but I don't know why it wouldn't be."

"Cool, thanks!"

Turning back to the night nurse, I say, "There, problem solved. Go ahead and give me report on him. Kelly isn't going to care."

She looks frantic as she speaks, a state I am all too familiar with being in at the end of a hectic shift. "O.K., so this is Bart. He came in originally for a GI bleed, which stopped at some point but has since restarted. They took him to surgery in the middle of the night because they believed he had a perforated bowel. They thought they had cauterized the bleed while they were in there, but he's still shitting blood. His blood pressure has been unstable ever since he got back, and he hasn't produced more than thirty cc of urine in the last two days, so they want to start CVVHD today. He's also been super confused since he got back from surgery. Like I said, he keeps calling me the devil. I think he's hallucinating. He says he doesn't want CVVHD, but I don't think he's in the right state of mind to refuse care. I don't know. Here's my report sheet, and my cell number. I'm back tonight, but feel free to text me if you have any questions. If I forgot to tell you anything, hopefully it's on this sheet, but it's really not a bother if you need to reach out."

She hands me a piece of paper full of notes and vital signs and writes her cell phone number in one of its corners in red ink. I'm familiar with feeling personally responsible for the outcome of a patient who isn't doing well after having spent an entire shift trying and failing to turn their condition around. I too have given my cell phone number to the nurse I've passed report to in case I forgot pertinent information while giving report, or in case there's any way I can help from home. It's hard to say why we feel this responsibility for some patients and not others, but I'm sure all nurses do. I feel like it happens when the patient's situation has gotten so complicated and has so many details that we're afraid the next nurse will miss one and it will cost the patient their life.

Kelly and Diane come down to meet us just as the night nurse hands me the paper. "Hey," Kelly says, "I don't know why they gave him to Diane instead of you, but I'm sure she can figure it out and just ask you for help as needed. We don't have any helper nurses today, so you'll need to help each other anyway."

"Yeah . . ." Diane begins tentatively, "I mean I'm sure I can figure it out. I've just never done it before. And I know those patients are usually pretty unstable."

"Well, this patient is technically PCU status," Kelly says. "He's not even on any oxygen."

"Yeah," I say, "but they're going to have to change his status to ICU if they start CVVHD. Plus, he's on pressers now. I don't mind helping, but it's kind of unfair to have to care for and chart on two patients *plus* teach and manage a CVVHD. I'd much rather just take the CVVHD and help Diane with the more stable patients."

Kelly sighs. "Yeah, O.K. But I think they wanted you open to take any admit. It's just you two working over here. Are you sure you're O.K. taking this patient knowing you might also get an admit?"

"Yeah, it's fine," I reply. "I might not even get one."

"O.K.. Well, you two let Andrew or me know if you need help. We're charging today." Thank goodness. With those two in charge, even the worst shift can be bearable.

My other patient is a Jewish man on a trach due to COVID. I'm told during report that he doesn't speak, but he gets very upset if anyone tries to take his Torah out of his hands. Occupational Therapy has been trying to work with him to improve his breathing enough to wean him off the vent so he can be downgraded to a long-term care facility. Every time I go in to turn him, I first have to promise I'm not taking his Torah. But, considering it takes most of his energy to breathe, he ends up being a fairly low-maintenance patient.

I head into Bart's room to do my morning assessment and start with four questions I haven't been able to ask my patients in a while.

"What is your name and birthday?"

He answers correctly.

"Where are we right now?"

"The hospital."

"Why are you here?"

"They keep doing things to me, but nothing seems to stop this dang bleed. I'm sick and tired of it! And that girl last night, she is *not* to be trusted. That's why I wouldn't answer these questions for her."

O.K., not entirely rational, but he's answering the questions correctly.

"And what year is it?"

Not only does he answer with 2020, but he gives me the exact month and day as well. Typically, patients give me the full date when they can tell I don't trust that they know it and they want to assure me that they do.

"O.K., excellent. Well, Bart, do you understand that they want to start dialysis on you today? You haven't been producing enough urine on your own, and they're hoping dialysis will help regulate your blood pressure a little better."

"I don't understand what peeing has to do with my blood pressure, but I'm not interested. They told me that surgery was going to fix things, and if it didn't, then it's time for me to meet Jesus. I don't want any more doctors in here, and I don't want any dialysis. I want to meet my Lord and savior Jesus Christ!"

Oh my. I need more coffee. "O.K., well, the doctor will be in in a little bit to talk with you about all this," I say as I leave the room, ignoring Bart's continued protests against seeing more doctors.

When the doctors arrive, Bart gives them the same spiel he gave me: if the surgery didn't fix all of his problems, then the Lord is calling him home. "But we didn't think surgery *would* fix all your problems," the physician tells him, sounding as exasperated as I feel. "Surgery fixed one problem—your perforated bowels. Your body has other problems that need to be fixed in other ways."

"I don't want any more fixin's. I just want to be left alone to meet my Lord and savior Jesus Christ!"

"But sir," the physician tries again, "you're not *that* sick. We can help you. We can fix these problems and get you out of here."

"I'm in the ICU, aren't I? You can't tell me I'm not sick if I'm in the ICU!"

The physician leaves the room and beckons me to follow. In the hallway, he tells me that he's going to defer this issue to the nephrologist, who will hopefully be able to do a better job of explaining to Bart that he isn't actively dying, and that dialysis will be helpful for his current condition. In the meantime, I'm supposed to maintain his vital signs with the medications we already have running and try to convince him to let me give him his morning meds.

This is a moral issue I frequently run into as an ICU nurse. Patients get tired of fighting, and they're often close enough to death that giving up will kill them. Patients refuse their medications without proper understanding of what they're doing, yet legally and ethically I cannot force them to consent to any treatments they are not willing to try. I feel caught in the crossfire of the physicians and patients. Technically, I work for neither, but ethically I am struggling to decide who ultimately gets more say in the matter.

"O.K.," I say. "But he has the right to refuse his medications. He's lucid as far as I can tell, and I'm not going to force him to take anything if he's adamant that he doesn't want it."

After speaking with the nephrologist, Bart still does not want to do dialysis. The nephrologist tells me to set it up anyway, and at that request, my mind settles on who I'm serving. "The patient does not want it," I say "He's adamant about that. He's lucid. He has a right to refuse treatment regardless of our medical opinions and suggestions. I'm not going to force treatment onto a person telling me they do not want it. That is assault."

I'm pissed. I'm so tired of having these types of conversations. *The family doesn't understand the torture they're putting the patient through,* or *The patient's will specifically said they didn't want this,* or *The patient says he wants comfort care, so we are morally obligated to let him die in peace.* It's exhausting. Many people think the hardest part of my job is witnessing so much death and trauma. But it's not. The hardest part is watching patients suffer unnecessarily—and extensively—at the behest of their loved one's inability to let them go or their physician's inability to see them as an actual, suffering human being with thoughts and opinions independent from their medically acclaimed ones. I am constantly forced into in the roles of "middleman" and "moral compass" and "unbiased, objective third party," and these are the cases that get my panties in a wad at work and keep me up at night. It's hard to know whether I'm fighting for the right thing, but my gut is often lit aflame telling me that I am—and that I need to fight harder.

At around 1 p.m., one of Bart's family members arrives to visit. When I share the good news with Bart, he screams, "No! No visitors! They'll only try to convince me to live. They wouldn't understand. I don't want to see anyone but my Lord and Savior Jesus Christ today."

Oh boy. "Bart," I say softly, "they came all this way and waited in that big line outside the hospital to see you. Surely you can spare just ten minutes for them?" My bargaining goes nowhere with Bart, so I get Andrew to see whether maybe he can speak some magic. He cannot. In fact, Bart seems *more* adamant about not having visitors after speaking with Andrew. Somehow, though, the resident manages to talk him into allowing a short visit.

His niece sits with him for a little while, and he seems genuinely glad to see her. He tells her that he's made up his mind to meet Jesus later today. I do my best to explain to his niece everything that's going on. "Since he's fully lucid, he's allowed to refuse any and all treatments. The doctors want to try dialysis, so we're getting the machine ready to run, but we can't administer it against his will."

His niece seems tearful as she nods. I find a chair for her and set it beside Bart's bed. While they chat, I get the CVVHD machine hooked up and ready to go as instructed. I still don't feel comfortable starting it, though.

I eat lunch while Bart's niece is still here to keep him company. When I get back, I'm told she's gone home for the day, so it's time to start CVVHD.

"But Bart still doesn't want it," I say.

"I know, babe," Kelly says, "but the nephrologist still isn't convinced he's lucid enough to make that call. He wants you to start it. You're within your license to question and disagree with him, but ultimately he gets the final say."

"I'll start it," I say grudgingly, "but I'm not happy about it."

"I know. I'm here if you need me." With that, Kelly goes back towards the front of the unit, and I'm left to hook up the CVVHD.

Luckily, Bart has drifted off to sleep. I turn the lights off in his room and do my best to get the dialysis machine running without waking him up. Success. Once it's running and I've charted my disagreement with starting it, I head off to find the resident. I reiterate that I disagree about starting CVVHD. "He hasn't sounded confused or answered one question wrong all morning," I remind her. "He's completely with it, and he doesn't want this treatment. It's technically assault to be giving it to him against his will. I don't like it. I know our job is to save people, but if they want to die, it's our job to respect that wish, too."

"I hear you," the resident tells me. "I think the nephrologist is just having a hard time with that because this guy isn't actively dying. We can still save him."

"I know, but if we don't do CVVHD, he'll probably be dead in a week. And that's what he wants. I know that as healthcare providers we want to save people, but sometimes the gracious thing is to let them go. We didn't get into medicine to torture people against their will, and that's essentially what we're doing by putting him on CVVHD."

"I'll see what I can do. I'm sorry, this nephrologist can be particularly difficult to persuade. But I'll do my best. I agree with you."

"Thank you," I tell her. "And it must be a nephrologist thing. All of the ones I worked with back home were the same way. Very particular." We laugh and I go to check on Bart.

The physicians were right; after an hour of CVVHD, I'm able to turn off the small amount of pressers I'd had Bart on. He wakes up when I go to disconnect the IV drip from his central line. "WHAT ARE YOU DOING TO ME?" he shouts, startling me.

"Hey hey hey," I tell him in as soothing a voice as I can manage. "It's O.K. I'm just disconnecting the medications we had you on. Like you wanted." I show him that the IV tubing is no longer attached to his central line.

"Good." he says. "Then get this thing out of me." he points towards his central line.

"Bart, I can't. It's not up to me whether or not that can come out. It's up to your doctors, and they don't want me to remove it. You might need it."

"I don't need any of this shit to meet my Lord and Savior! Get it off. I want to meet him in peace."

"I understand, Bart, but again, it isn't up to me. I could lose my job if I took that line out without your doctor's permission. You don't want that, do you?"

Usually, this guilt trip manages to get patients off my back, and Bart is no different. He remains unhappy, though. "Well, then get that bastard in here and have him take it out himself. I'm fixing to meet my maker."

"O.K., I'll get right on that. In the meantime, just try to go back to sleep." I turn to leave before he can say anything else. *For someone who wants to meet Jesus today, he sure is swearing a lot.*

After much pleading from Bart's resident, the nephrologist agrees to come see Bart, along with his primary attending and a psychiatrist, to determine whether or not Bart really is competent enough to decide to die. After spending thirty minutes in his room listening to him answer all the psychiatrist's questions correctly and yell multiple times that this is all ridiculous and that they need to "get this shit off of me and leave me in peace to meet Jesus," the three physicians exit his room and tell me to do what Bart wants.

Predictably, the nephrologist throws a fit about it first. "I guess we're in the killing business now. The one patient we can save, and he doesn't even want to live. I can't understand the point of surgery and all the other shit we've done for him if he ultimately just wants to die. He's not going to die overnight. I don't know why he thinks that. I don't know why I bother." He says this more to himself than anyone around him. I can sympathize. I prefer to save people, too. But more than that, I prefer to abide by their individual wishes, and this is Bart's. It's not my job or my right to push my wishes onto my patients. It *is* my job to advocate for what they want, and Bart wants to die. While I agree that he probably won't die overnight, I imagine he'll pass in a few days without dialysis and antibiotics.

The shift is nearly over. I've spent the last eleven hours trying to get Bart's care team to agree on this point. "O.K. Bart," I tell him as I enter his room, "let's get you unhooked from this machine." I return his blood from the dialysis machine back to his body. I ask whether he's comfortable, whether he wants any more pillows behind his head or at his sides.

"Yeah. Prop me up a little bit so I can see Jesus when he comes."

"Sure thing, Bart." I grab a pillow off the chair his niece was sitting on and ask him to turn slightly to his right so I can push it behind his back. When he turns, his sheets move with him, and I see a massive puddle of blood underneath his legs.

"Oh Bart!" I exclaim, setting the pillow back on the chair. "We need to get you cleaned up!"

"You don't need to do nothin' except let me be so I can meet my Maker!"

"No, seriously Bart. You've had some bloody stool. I can't let you sit here in it. Why didn't you tell me you needed to be changed?" I feel awful. I have no idea how long he's been lying like this.

"I don't need nothin'. Let me be!"

"Bart, don't you want to be nice and clean when Jesus comes to see you later?" Sometimes bargaining a patient's story against them works. I feel like that's all I've done today: bargain. Bargain with Bart to resume treatment, to see his family. Bargain with his physicians to stop treatment, to abide by his wishes. I'm exhausted, and it's almost time to go. I cannot leave him like this, and I'm running out of patience for the day.

"He loves me just the way I am," Bart says. "I don't need nothin'."

I sigh.

"Hey, Andrew," I say when I spot him in the hallway. "Could you please help me clean up Bart? He's had some bloody stool. He doesn't want to be cleaned up, so I might need a little manpower to get him to cooperate. I can't leave him like this."

"Sure thing, Laura. I'll be right there." Andrew leaves to get bedding supplies so we can get Bart changed.

We tell Bart what we're going to do, and I make it clear that it's not optional. "If you wan to meet Jesus, that's your prerogative. But you do not get to meet your night-shift nurse in a pile of your own bloody stool. Understand?" Against Bart's screaming protests, we flatten his bed out and Andrew forces his body to turn towards him so I can wipe his backside.

"Unhand me! Unhand me you sinner! I WILL CURSE YOU! YOU WILL BE JUDGED BY THE LORD ALMIGHTY!" At this Bart reaches up and bites Andrew on the shoulder, who understandably drops him back onto the bed.

"BART!" we both yell at once.

"That is NOT O.K.!" I say in my most stern mom-voice, pointing a finger in his face. Exasperation and irritation seep through. "We are trying to help you. You may not sit in filth for the remainder of your life. I won't allow it. Now I have done a lot for you today, and I do not appreciate you harming my friend. I need you to cooperate. I need you to let us help you. And we *do not* bite. Am I clear?"

"Let me get Kelly," Andrew says, heading out the door. "We need more hands."

Bart is still screaming obscenities when Kelly and Andrew return together. Andrew puts Kelly up by Bart's head and warns her what happened moments ago, and with the two of them holding him still I'm able to wipe off the remaining dried blood from his backside and get a set of clean sheet underneath him. They continue holding his arms at his sides as

I change him into a new gown. They pull him into the most comfortable-looking position we can manage with him squirming against us, and then we leave his room and let him continue screaming at nothing.

"Thanks a lot, Laura, now I'm going to be judged," Andrew says jokingly as we head up to the front of the unit together. We're all dying laughing at Bart's "curse".

"Well, there comes a time for all of us!" I say between giggles. "Thanks for your help, guys."

As the night-shift nurses trickle in, I watch for the one who gave me report on Bart this morning. She said she'd be back tonight, and I'm grateful because I don't know that I have the energy to explain everything that's happened with Bart in the last couple days in detail to someone new. But she never comes, and when I say something about it to the night charge, a friend of hers overhears and says, "Oh yeah, she called in. Said she couldn't emotionally handle Bart's case two nights in a row."

Poor thing. I totally get that. I explain everything as best as I can to the nurse who takes him. I give her the report sheet that was given to me earlier this morning, but first I tear off the previous nurse's phone number. On my way home, I shoot her a text to let her know that Bart has decided to be on comfort care per his and his family's wishes. She texts back right away, thanking me for the info.

That night I drift off to sleep wondering whether Bart will be there when I return tomorrow.

Bart is still there come the next day, and I have miraculously been given two new patients since comfort care measures do not require ICU skills. A lot of times that sort of thing will get my panties in a wad, because I often feel connected to and responsible for a patient I treated who is now passing, but after all of the rigmarole with Bart yesterday, I am thankful for the break. The patients I've been assigned to are in the same hallways as Bart's room, so I let his nurse know to holler at me if she has any questions or needs any help. Come midday she takes me up on that offer.

"The patient's niece says that yesterday our manager approved for both her and her mom to come visit today, but apparently our manager didn't let the front desk people know, so they're not letting them both in."

"Are you freaking kidding me? He's dying! Ugh, I'll handle it. Watch my patients for me." I stomp to the front of the unit, where Bart's niece looks tearful and concerned.

"Hi," she says, relief flooding her face when she sees me. "They wouldn't let my mom in downstairs. They said there's still only one visitor at a time, but your manager said she would make a special exception considering the circumstances. Except this gal said your manager isn't here today. I don't know what to do."

"Yeah," I tell her, "they don't work weekends. Don't worry, I'll get her in."

I storm down to the front of the hospital where I find Bart's sister standing near the entrance looking as tearful as her daughter did. "Hi," I say as I approach. "You must be Bart's sister! Let me handle this." I cut the line of other visitors waiting to be checked in. "Hi," I shout to one of the secretaries in my no-nonsense voice. "I work in the ICU upstairs. I'm taking care of a patient on comfort care, and yesterday our manager approved for both his niece and his sister to visit him today."

"O.K.," she says warily. "And who are you?"

"I'm Laura. Laura Luther. ICU nurse," I say, thrusting my badge up to her window. "This woman's brother is dying. You need to let her up to say goodbye."

After discussing this in hushed tones with another secretary, whose facial expression seems to say she couldn't care less if we were letting an elephant up to the unit, she takes down my name and employee I.D. and tells me that if my manager in fact did not approve this yesterday, it will be on me.

"Fine. Thank you," I respond curtly. I take Bart's sister up to the unit.

As Bart's nurse and I place two chairs on either side of his bed, she informs his niece and sister that he's been sleeping most of the day. We leave them alone with him, and I become engrossed in caring for my own patients, feeling happy and slightly self-righteous that I was here today to help make this family visit happen.

Towards the end of the shift, Kelly, who's charging again today, comes up to me and says, "Get a load of this! Bart, that guy you worked so hard to get on comfort care yesterday, has decided to resume treatment. Says he thought he'd die by now and if he hasn't then it must be the Father's will for him to live. Can you believe it?"

I literally cannot believe it. I also cannot stop banging my head against the wall at the news. I put *so* much effort into making Bart's wish for comfort care come true yesterday. And now his efforts at surviving his current conditions are nearly twenty-four hours behind what they would've been had I been able to start CVVHD the day before, thus rendering his not-amazing odds of survival even less amazing. *Thank you, Father, that I'm off tomorrow and will no longer have to deal with this shit.* I guess Bart and I have both faith and the use of swear-words in common.

CALL ME PRINCESS

THE FIRST DAY OF THE last week of my contract is a good one. Or at least, it's supposed to be. Aside from the fact that I'm beyond ecstatic that I'll be flying home at the end of the week, today is my last shift with Arina, and I'm looking forward to working with her. Which is why I become infuriated when I arrive to my unit and am told, "They're sending you to Main ICU."

"What?" I say, half-panicked. "The nursing office told me to come here!"

"Well I don't know what to tell you," the night-shift charge nurse tells me. "They told me they were sending you to Main ICU."

I set my stuff down and power walk up to the nursing office to ask for my unit assignment, something I stopped doing after the first two weeks of working here, since they told me I'd more than likely be assigned to the sixth-floor unit for the remainder of my contract. I hold my breath as the office clerk searches for my name on her list. I let out a huge exhale when she tells me "Sixth floor."

I storm back to my unit, heart pounding. I'm going anywhere. "I asked them again," I tell the night shift charge, "and they said I'm assigned to *this* unit."

"I know you were," she tells me, letting out a sigh. "But Main ICU is short, so we have to send one of you to them."

"O.K. Well, I'm not going." I say, crossing my arms and trying to stand tall. "I'll just go home." I remembered Leah telling me that she said this to the nursing office clerk on her last day when they had tried to send her to her least favorite unit, and they folded and sent somebody else. I hope it will work for me, too.

The night shift charge sighs again. "Okay, hang on." She dials the phone and starts talking exasperatedly to someone on the other line.

I feel bad. I'm sure this headache is the last thing she wants to deal with at the end of what was surely a long night. But I tell myself to stand my ground. I've been through a lot of shit these past twelve weeks. I'm determined to make this final week a good one. I feel even worse when Kelly walks in and receives an update on the situation. She looks at me questioningly.

"I'm not going," I say to her when the night shift charge is done explaining.

"You might not have a choice, babe," she tells me.

"Sure I do. I'll just go home." I shrug. I sense that Kelly can see the regret in my eyes as I say this to her, but I have to stand firm. If I'm just bluffing, I'll look like an idiot.

After a minute of staring me down Kelly shrugs and says, "Well, it's your contract."

"It's my last week. I'll survive without the money."

"Good luck getting a new contract with that attitude."

I can't help but laugh. "I don't want a new contract. I want to go home. And I want to work here with Arina today. It's our last day together." I try to change my expression from defiant to puppy-dog pleading.

After some conversation between Kelly and the night charge, they tell Stephanie, another travel nurse on my unit, that she'll have to go to Main ICU today. "But the nursing office told me to come here!" she responds. I hold my breath.

"I know," Kelly tells her, "but they're short a nurse and we have to send somebody. I'm sorry."

Stephanie sighs but doesn't argue as she grabs her things to leave. I exhale. My heart is pounding out of my chest.

"You got lucky. I was prepared to call your bluff," Kelly tells me.

I smile and say, "Guess we'll never know how serious I was," as I walk off to find Arina.

She's beaming. She watched the whole thing play out. "I'm so proud of you," she whispers to me as I sit down next to her. "I've never seen you stand up for yourself like that before. How does it feel?"

"It was scary, but it honestly feels really good."

"I can imagine. That was amazing."

"I wasn't going to work on a different unit from you on our last day together."

She smiles at me, and we get to work. I'm assigned to care for Selena and Byron again, possibly the two most depressing patients on the unit. I had them for half the previous week, too. They've both been here for seemingly forever.

Byron has been a COVID patient on our unit since the day I touched ground in New York: April 17. By the time my contract is ending, he will have been a patient for ninety-two days. He's been intubated, extubated, and re-intubated. He's been on and off pressers, on and off CVVHD. The physicians won't trach him or do CVVHD anymore, because his prognosis is so poor, but they aren't pushing for the family to withdraw care, either. His body is literally rotting away. Pieces of skin on his lower legs fall off each time I change the bandages on his shin wounds, which needs to be done three or four times per shift due to the amount of bodily fluids seeping out of them. He has another wound on his coccyx that has to be changed and repacked once per shift. He opens his eyes, but he doesn't really look at anything. No one knows whether he can still see. He can't move anything on his body, so we have to turn him every two hours and hope that he's comfortable. Right now, he requires Levo to keep his blood pressure up and an IV medication called Bumex to make him pee. He seems more dead than alive to me, and every time I provide nursing care to him, it feels like I'm torturing him instead of helping. I can't help but think, *This is not why I got into nursing.*

Sandra is just as depressing. She has a mental delay of some sort, so no one is really sure how much she understands what's going on and what we're doing for her, to her. She's been intubated and extubated a lot, too. I remember caring for her her first week here. She wasn't intubated then, but she was still a very busy patient. She has extreme weakness in her arms and legs, so she has to be frequently repositioned, too. Her eyes constantly express pain, but she doesn't speak, and I'm never quite sure whether I've made things better or worse for her. Her heart likes to randomly go into A-fib RVR, a dangerous arrhythmia that can quickly become lethal if not medically treated. She has a trach and requires the ventilator to breath. She's not on any cardiac drips at the moment, but she's on several IV antibiotics, fluids, and tube feeds. She's very pale colored, and her face possesses a constant expression of pain or weariness. She kind of looks the way a dog's eyes do when you tell him something he doesn't want to hear; unhappy, but unable to do anything about it. Sandra also requires frequent changes of her several wound dressings. Her entire body is swollen, and various parts of her are weeping bodily fluids throughout the day.

It's nearly 10 a.m. when I go into Byron's room to give him his morning meds. An attending I've never met is looking at him when I walk in, and he immediately starts asking me questions about Byron without so much as a "good morning" or "how do you do." I answer them as best as I can as I set down the various medications and supplies I've brought in with me. He asks me whether I can place an order for a different medication to try and get Byron to pee more. "I can't," I tell him, beginning to wonder whether he knows I'm a nurse, "but I'm sure your resident could enter that for you."

"Which resident is covering Byron today?"

"I'm not sure. I haven't looked yet."

He pauses what he's doing and looks at me with scolding eyes. "You don't know the name of your resident?" he asks. "What would you do if there was an emergency?"

I shrug and tell him, "I'd just walkie *resident to fifty-nine* and one would show up." He starts to leave the room as he continues talking, so I follow him out. "That is entirely unacceptable. You should *always* know your residents name," he scoffs as he turns to walk down the hall.

"O.K.," I holler after him. He stops and halfway turns back towards me. I can tell by his expression that he wasn't expecting a response. "Well, when you get to the residents' lounge and you figure out who's covering Byron today," I continue, "why don't you ask him or her what *my* name is? I have a feeling they don't know. I have a feeling *you* don't know, either." I also have a feeling no one has ever had the balls to talk back to this physician, because he doesn't respond. He just walks away. Like I said, it's my last week. I don't have a lot left to lose, and physicians don't sign my paycheck.

Between the never-ending dressing changes, Arina and I make the most out of our last workday together. We cry from laughing as I reenact my encounter with the attending. We make Instagram stories of ourselves dancing to random songs, including one to "Hot in Here" where we seductively strip off one piece of PPE at a time for the camera. We shop online together. We talk about everything and nothing, just like we always do. Neither of our patients have medical emergencies today, a welcome rarity.

When the end of the day comes, I feel a slight sadness, but Arina will have none of it. "Today is not goodbye," she tells me. "We'll spend all of Friday together, so today is just 'see you later.'"

I know she's right, but I'm still sad. Days working with Arina were some of the best I had, and today has been no exception.

The next day I get the same patients: Sandra and Byron. My friend Gage is my helper-nurse, which is good, because my day ends up being very busy. Sandra is a mess. It's as if she rotted overnight. I mean, she didn't look very good the day before, but she didn't look this close to what I imagine aliens looking like, either. Her skin tone is that of a ghost, and her veins are popping out deep purple on her face like the little girl in *The Exorcist*. I observe this to Gage as we leave her room after getting report from her night nurse.

"I realized a long time ago that ICU nursing is simply disgusting," he replies. "All these patients have shit coming out of their butts, wounds weeping God-knows-what out of God-knows-where, and never-ending secretions coming out of their breathing tube." "You're not wrong," I reply, "but most patients aren't *that* gross. I swear she didn't look quite this bad yesterday." I have a bad feeling about what that means for the rest of my shift.

Somehow, just as we're starting the Levo, Sandra's midline goes bad. "You've got to be fucking kidding me!" I scream. I page the PA to Sandra's room. "I need a new line in room fifty-eight stat!" I try in vain to find somewhere to stick an IV, but Sandra's body is puffy everywhere. "Do you know whether we maybe have an IO starter somewhere?" I ask Gage, who clearly does not know what to do right now.

"A what?" he asks, looking more lost.

"Never mind."

"Hey, I'm here," says the PA as she enters the room. "We need a central line for her so we can start Levo, right?"

"Well," I say, "I officially don't even have an IV. Her midline is shit. I don't know what happened to it. We've been using it all day."

"Fuck—really?" She looks as stressed as I feel. "Have you been able to get an IV?"

"I literally see nothing. Except maybe these purple veins in her forehead," I say, only half-joking.

"Yeah, you're right. O.K., maybe I can start an EJ to hold us over until I can get a central line placed. I'll need you to hold her head in place for me, though."

"Yeah, no problem," I tell her. Except it is sort of a problem, because Sandra's neck is as swollen as the rest of her body, making it difficult to simultaneously turn her neck and keep her ventilator intact with her trach.

I send Gage to check on Byron since I doubt he'll be much help in here—there's really no room for all of us anyway; Sandra very well may be in the smallest room on the unit—and then I pull Sandra's bed away from the wall so I can stand behind it and hold her head in place. I have to climb up on the back of the bed in order to even reach her head with her body tilted up at ninety degrees. I can't see her full blood pressure on the monitor, but I decide it doesn't matter. I can see her heart rate, and there's really nothing I can do other than compressions without an IV. Luckily, all of this moving around seems to be agitating Sandra enough to keep her blood pressure at a reasonable level.

As she begins to work, the PA informs me that the resident is busy calling Sandra's family. He's attempting to explain to them just how bad her condition is and hopefully persuade them towards making Sandra comfort care. "Do you think someone could get the central-line kit set up while I fuck with placing this EJ?"

"Sure," I tell her. I use the walkie-talkie to ask whether anyone can heed her request.

Andrew soon pops his head into our room. "Hey, so, what do you guys need?"

"I need a central-line kit," the PA says. "As soon as I can manage an EJ, I need to try to get the central line placed. I also need an ART line setup and some fluids."

"Yeah . . ." Andrew hesitates. "The residents usually do all that."

"Well does it *look* like I have a resident in here helping me? Laura can't move until I get an EJ placed, and this patient needs a central line, an ART line, and some Levophed. Pronto!"

I give Andrew an apologetic look. "I'll be back," he says, popping his head back out.

"I mean, sorry to be a bitch," the PA says to herself as much as to me, "but is that seriously too much to ask? We're obviously fucking busy in here."

"Yeah, I'm sorry," I tell her. "I don't really get that either." After a pause, I say, "At the last hospital I worked at in Kansas City, we didn't have residents, so the nurses were expected to do the setup *and* assist on all line placements for our patients. It's just a different world here."

"Wow, really? I feel like here I can't even get a nurse to bring me supplies."

"Yeah . . ." I say.

After what feels like an hour, the PA finally manages to get an EJ. Around the same time that we get Sandra hooked up to Levo again, the resident comes in. "Hey," I just got off the phone with Sandra's family. They aren't on board with straight-up comfort care, but they *are* starting to understand that we're running out of things to do for her, so they said not to escalate her care anymore than we currently have."

"Great," says the PA, sounding slightly jaded and looking at me. "Then I don't need to place anymore lines and she doesn't need to be started on Levo."

"Got it," I reply.

The PA leaves with the resident, so now it's just me and Sandra in the room.

I turn off the IV pump I had been priming to start. Sandra's next blood pressure reading shows a significant drop from her previous ones. Her time has come; I can feel it.

"O.K. Sandra," I say, looking her in the eyes (although that she's actually looking back at me is highly unlikely). "Your family understands. It's O.K., O.K.? You can let go now. They don't need you to fight anymore. They love you very much, and I'm here with you. But you need to go now, O.K.? Because if you don't go before my shift ends, I can't promise someone will be here with you when you die. I have no idea how long your doctors will let you live like this, and you *cannot* live like this, O.K.? Do you hear me? It's time to go, Sandra. I'm right here." I hold her hand and stare at her monitor. Her heart rate holds steady for a while, but each blood pressure reading is lower than the last. Within fifteen minutes, she's gone. I do not cry. The silence of Sandra's room feels ill-suited to emotion, as if it does not want to be penetrated.

I turn off her monitor and her ventilator, tell her thank you, and leave her room. I pass the PA on my way back to the physician's room. "She's dead," I tell her.

"Not my problem now," she says as she continues to walk off the unit.

I strut down to the physician's room and open the door. "Sandra's dead. Room fifty-eight."

"Who pronounced her?" a resident asks.

"I guess I did. So—one of you will need to officially take care of that." I'm done for today. I feel stone cold, although I know there are feelings underneath just waiting for me to thaw.

As I walk out of the hospital and towards my Airbnb, I pass the PA that was in Sandra's room with me.

"Hey," she stops me. "I'm really sorry about what I said back there. It sounded heartless, and I didn't mean that." She wipes her hand across her face. "This is all just getting to me. I can't even understand why we let people like her live as long as we do. It feels like torture. I'm exhausted, and I don't feel like I made much of a difference today. Or ever."

My heart softens. I often feel this way myself, and I know we are all doing the best we can processing the constant loss of life around us.

"I understand," I say. "I try not to take anything here personally anymore."

She sighs in response. "I hate that I sometimes have to come off as a bitch to get things done, but I feel like I'm treated differently than some of the residents, and so I do act like a bitch to get things done."

"We have to do that sometimes," I agree. "And you are in the unique position of being both a woman and a physician's assistant in an environment full of multiple male residents and attendings who are primarily running the show in this medical program. Add to that a bunch of traveling nurses who have different perceptions of residents and PAs, and the fact that the world is on fire and everybody is dying, and you've got this hot mess. We're all just doing the best we can. And even pre-COVID I had my fair share of bitchy moments when I thought it would get me what my patients needed. It doesn't matter what anybody thinks of you. What matters is that you can sleep at night knowing you did everything you could to help your patients that day."

Nothing has ever made me appreciate the fact that we're all just human quite like this pandemic.

NINETY-TWO DAYS AND COUNTING

My last day feels anticlimactic. None of my friends are working today, so no one even knows it's my last shift without me telling them. I don't have a helper nurse, and Byron is my patient again. I'm thankful to have stable patients (the whole unit is fairly calm today); however, Byron has been here since day one of my contract and is currently more dead than he is alive, with no hope of his family moving towards comfort care anytime soon. It's fucking depressing.

I make sure his wounds get redressed twice throughout the shift, and in my downtime, I prepare for the interview I have scheduled the following day. There's a hospital in Kansas City with a Post Anesthesia Care Unit position open, and thanks to patient situations like Byron's, I am all too ready to start working in a different environment. I read the history page for the hospital, read various potential interview questions for a PACU nurse, and try to put my reasons for leaving the ICU into professional-sounding words.

I had an interview with that hospital's HR hiring manager the week before, and it went really well. I explained to her that I had never intended to be a travel nurse; I had just felt called to help in NYC. Now that I have helped, I'm ready to come home and eager to learn something new. I didn't tell the HR rep this, but I truly feel that I have paid my dues in the ICU.

When I graduated nursing school, I thought I would be in the ICU forever. I also thought I would go back to school to become a certified nurse anesthetist. Now, though, the thought of either of those things makes me want to puke. I can't imagine working one more ICU shift, and I definitely can't imagine going back to school so soon. I'm barely managing to get myself to work this shift. And if I'm being *really* honest, I've barely managed to make myself work for the past three weeks: It's all just become so depressing.

What started as a wild adventure in the midst of nonstop chaos has become a never-ending drudgery caring for patients, like Byron, who are more dead than alive thanks to a fight against COVID. While Byron has lost the fight little by little over the past thirteen weeks, I have lost patients left and right to this disease. To see that, after so much loss and heartache, this *still* isn't over is disheartening. And to see that after all this time we are still letting patients like Byron suffer . . . I just can't be a part of that suffering anymore.

I want to help people—that's why I got into nursing. I can count the people I've saved from COVID-19 on one hand; meanwhile I lost track of all the lives I've lost *months* ago, and I haven't even been fighting this virus for half a year. It's devastating to watch people live knowing full well that we have done—are doing—everything we can for them, and it's not enough. It's devastating to watch people live through rotting flesh and breathing tubes and feeding tubes *well* past the point that they should have been let go, past the point that they should have found peace, past the point that they should have stopped feeling pain. I did not get into nursing to cause pain, and yet with patients like Byron, who is eighty years old and has been intubated for several months and probably already has permanent brain damage as a result, that's essentially what I'm doing. There is often pain and suffering in the continuation of human life.

PACU seems like an opportunity for a new beginning. An opportunity to help people again. Patient's come in for surgery, they get fixed, we (the PACU nurses) give them medication to help make the pain go away, and then we send them on their merry way, slightly better off than they were when they came in that morning. Sounds perfect. Sign me up.

Towards the end of the shift, I get a call from my travel nurse recruiter. I'm in the middle of one of Byron's dressing changes, so I don't pick up. "Congratulations, Laura!" she says at the start of the voicemail. "You've been offered an extension at your current hospital. Call me right away to confirm that you'd like this extension. Congratulations again on getting what you wanted!"

I laugh out loud.

At the beginning of my contract, I *had* wanted to extend it. I told my recruiter this weekly for the first two months. I had friends, I liked the focus on patient care over charting specifics, I liked my Airbnb, I liked the money that was rolling in, and July had felt like light-years away, so moving the end-date to August hadn't seemed like a big deal. Plus, I though ensuring my recruiter I'd be interested in an extension would help prevent my contract from getting cut short (a common occurrence when hospitals over-hire for a crisis). But now? Congratulations? Yeah, right. If the hospital didn't wanted me to stay before, they can't have me now. Too little, too late. I have a one-way ticket to Kansas City dated two days from today, and I have every intention of getting on that plane. Even if they offered me double the money (I didn't ask what they were offering, but if I had to guess, they're probably offering less than what I currently make), I wouldn't take it. New York felt like home within minutes of my arriving. Now, all I want is to leave.

The phone interview with the Kansas City PACU director doesn't go as well as the one with the HR manager did. The director sounds busy and tired from the moment she says hello, and five minutes into our conversation she has to hang up because a patient in her department is having a heart attack. I try not to panic as I pack and repack my two giant suitcases, my preparation notes from the day before spread all over my bed so I can read any of them at a moment's notice.

What little luggage room I regained by using up my toiletries has been overtaken by books I found on the sidewalks of Brooklyn (one of my favorite things about the city: people will just leave books they don't want any more on their front stoop). I haven't had time to read them all, and I desperately want to take a piece of the city home with me. I end up leaving half of them behind after several failed attempts at zipping my suitcases. I'm definitely not going to be under the weight limit for luggage no matter what I do, and this time around I'm repacking not to get one suitcase under fifty pounds, but simply to make everything fit.

I'm nearly done packing when the director calls back. "Thanks again for being so flexible," she tells me.

"Flexibility is just one of many traits that would make me an excellent candidate for this position . . ." I begin.

About an hour later, we get off the phone. The position sounds perfect for me, and I say a quick prayer that I'll get it, knowing that that decision is now out of my hands. I check the time. I have about two hours before I need to be at Arina's. *Shit. I have to mail this painting.*

I get dressed, throw a mask over my face, and grab the oversized painting of the Chrysler building that I had bought in the park the day of my fifteen-mile run. It's far too big to carry onto the plane, and I needed to make sure it gets home in one protected piece. Aside from the books I've picked up, it's the only thing I've bought myself to commemorate this experience. I search for the nearest post office on my phone and see that it's about a mile away. Three blocks into the walk there, my entire body is sweaty from holding the painting. It isn't heavy, per say, but it is awkwardly wide, forcing me to hold it out from my body at a strange angle that makes my arms sore. It's a hot mid-July day, and there isn't a lot of shade coverage on the way.

The line for the post office is out the door of the building, and only when I get to the front of it thirty minutes later am I told that they don't sell any type of protective shipping boxes or coverings big enough for my painting. "Maybe you could try the UPS down the street?" the postal worker tells me. I feel optimistic about this, until the UPS cashier tells me the same thing and suggests I try the USPS.

I let out a haughty sigh. "I *just came* from the USPS store," I say between gritted teeth. "They suggested I come *here*."

"Well, I'm sorry, ma'am, but I don't know what to tell you. None of our boxes are tall enough to hold that painting."

I check my watch. I don't have time to try to find a third store. "Do you sell bubble wrap? Or packing paper? And tape?" I ask.

"Yeah, right over there." The cashier points to the back wall of the store.

"Perfect. I'll take it. I'll just wrap this thing up really well and then you can ship it."

"Well," he says, apprehension in the edge of his voice, "we still can't ship it."

"Why not?" I ask. Demand, really.

"Well, we only ship boxes. And we stack them all in the truck on top of each other. That painting would just get added to the pile and it would get smushed. We can't ship it."

"Can't I just write 'fragile' on it?"

"We don't ship fragile things unless they're in a box. That way we can put peanuts in the box to protect the items being shipped."

I can feel smoke threatening to come out of my ears. I started the week off with a limited number of marbles, and this shipping fiasco is taking the last one I have.

"FINE. Then I'll take the bubble wrap and the packing tape and the paper, and I'll wrap it myself and have the USPS ship it."

"Okay . . . but I really think your best bet would be to try another store."

"I don't have *time* to try another store. I'm getting on a plane *tomorrow*. This is my last night here, and I have somewhere to be in less than an hour, and I don't have a car, which means I've been walking this huge painting all over Brooklyn. I still have to pack, I still have to get ready for dinner tonight, and I NEED THIS PAINTING TO COME WITH

ME TO KANSAS CITY. I can't carry it onto the plane, so I NEED TO SHIP IT. Now. O.K.?"

Everyone in the store is staring at me at this point, but I don't have it in me to care. I pay for my packing supplies and then carry them and my painting to an aisle near the back and begin a very poor job of wrapping my painting like a package.

"Um, excuse me. Ma'am?" one of the other store clerks says to me.

"What?" I say tersely, not looking up from my project.

"This is the aisle we take passport photos in. I need to take a passport photo for this customer . . ." He winces as he points in a lady's direction.

Without speaking, I pick up my project and mov it one aisle over, where a different store clerk has the audacity to say, "That doesn't look like it's working out real well, little lady."

"WELL I DON'T HAVE ANY OTHER OPTIONS, DO I?" I snap, ripping a piece of tape off the roll as I speak. Moments later, he returns with some pieces of cardboard box.

"Perhaps these will help protect it in the front and back?" he offers in an apologetic and apprehensive tone.

"Yes. Thank you. These are helpful," I tell him with all the calmness of a serial killer.

It looks absolutely terrible, like a four-year-old has wrapped it, but when I'm done, the painting is completely covered with bubble wrap and cardboard, and I'm fairly confident that I've taped it all on there strongly enough to protect it during shipping. I've also written "fragile" in big capital letters all over the outer layer of packing paper. I'm prepared to pay extra to ship it this way, too.

I hold my head up high as I march my poorly wrapped package out of the UPS and back down the street towards the USPS, where I once again have to wait in a long line. Sweaty and exhausted, I attempt to catch my breath as I stand in line with my painting and text Arina an update on my ETA for dinner. The line is moving more quickly this time, and in the midst of my mental hurricane and frantic texting I'm shocked to hear a man bark at me "Six feet!"

I am so ready to go home.

With my painting packaged and sent off in the mail, and my suitcase sixty-five percent packed, I trek to the subway for one last ride to Arina's apartment. The day's stresses melt away the moment I see her.

"Hello, my sister!" she says as she guides me upstairs. "I have some things for you!"

"Oh wonderful! I have some things for you, too!" About a month ago, I purchased matching bracelets and rings in preparation for my departure. The words to describe just how much Arina's friendship and love has meant to me during my time here, and will continue to mean to me for the rest of my life, are difficult to convey. But based on her reaction to my goodbye card, I think I do a decent job.

I'll leave my words between us sisters, but I will share that the bracelets have a compass with two engraved leaves attached: one with an L, the other with an A. They came with compass rings, which I often wear on my right ring finger now to remind me that no matter what guy is or isn't in my life (or claiming my left ring finger), and no matter the distance between the two of us, I will always have my sister on my side.

As Arina opens her gift and reads her note, I play a Nahko and Medicine for the People song for her:

I'll be the earth that grounds you, from the chaos all around.

I'll be the home you return to; I can be your middle ground.
I will serve as a reminder, if you jump you will not fall.
Go on and spread those wings of reason; we are water after all.
. . .

A lighthouse when you're out to sea; a beacon when direction's all I
*   need.*
A compass if you know what I mean.
Drunk on that nectar of all that you are to me.

Afterwards, she takes me into her room and gives me beautiful dress after beautiful dress to try on and take home to keep. In those moments, I truly feel like her little sister. I could not be happier. You know you've found the most valuable type of person when time and the rest of the world cease to exist when you're with them.

Eventually, Arina's husband pops his head in to remind us that I came over for dinner. We go to a local eatery near their home, and it is the first time I have a meal at a restaurant, albeit outside, since my night out at Mission Taco with Brad several months ago. We order drinks and appetizers, we talk and laugh, and for a couple hours I forget all about the horrors of COVID and what they had done to this world, to my life, and to the many lives I've lost against it. All I know, and all I can focus on, are these beautiful people in front of me, and the crazy measures that life has gone to to bring us all together. If it means I get to keep Arina in my life and my heart forever, this wild journey has been worth it. She is a part of me now, just like all the other amazing nurses I've been privileged to work with, and all the patients I've been privileged to care for. They will all leave here with me in the morning, and a piece of my heart will stay behind in this city. This beautiful place I have come to call, and will continue to call, home.

In one of my favorite movies, *Garden State*, there's a line in which the main character is describing the feeling of being home and homesick and states, "It just sort of happens one day, one day and it's just gone. And you can never get it back. It's like you get homesick for a place that doesn't exist."

This is how I feel about New York. The New York I lived in was terrible and wonderful all at the same time, and no one else will ever experience it the way I did. I can't even recreate it if I wanted to. It is where I truly grew up. I had family. I had friends. I laughed. I cried. I ran. I explored. I was broken. I was healed.

After dinner, Arina and I go for a walk through the neighborhood at dusk. I chase several fireflies as we walk by the beautiful houses, reminding myself of when I was a little girl chasing fireflies in the yard on late summer evenings. We talk about everything and nothing. We dance, we run, we chase more fireflies. Eventually, we come to a grassy area and sit beneath a tree. We put on some music and continue to talk. I do some cartwheels—and quickly learn that my body is no longer young enough to do gymnastics without stretching first. We laugh. We lie on the grass together, looking up at the stars and listening to the music, both of us soaking in the final moments we have together. It's the perfect ending to a perfectly imperfect thirteen weeks in New York.

I blink and the next morning arrives. I finish packing all my things after I get ready. I do a couple more lookovers of the apartment. As I stand in the doorway, I take it in—this place I've called home for the past thirteen weeks. This place where I re-invented myself. This place where I watched so many lives pass through my own, like sand through my fingers at Coney Island Beach. This place where I healed some of the wounds caused by the loss of my Dad and my dog. This place where I grew so much, both as a nurse and as a person. I take one last look, one last breath, and close the door on this chapter of my life.

After hauling my fifty- and seventy-pound suitcases one by one down the two flights of stairs, I go back up and grab the box of things I'm going to leave behind. I lay out the books I've decided I can't bring with me, as well as my lunchbox, my mug, and my running shoes. I lay these things out on display the way I have seen so many others do over the course of my stay. Then, I call an Uber, and I'm off.

The check-in lady for Southwest is not as kind as the man in Kansas City, but I decide it doesn't matter. I've made enough money to afford to fly my luggage back for sixty dollars. On the plane, I can't focus. I'm so, so eager to get home. I listen to Nahko and Medicine for the People's albums, letting the lyrics soak into my soul as the east coast passes underneath me.

"I believe in the good things coming, coming, coming . . ."

The closer we get to Kansas City, the more I become aware of my left ring finger. I keep reaching down to twist my wedding ring, then remembering it isn't there—and hasn't been for months I haven't been wearing it since I first started caring for COVID patients in attempt to keep it clean and COVID-free. I ache to see Jake again. To see Rieger and Simba. My friends. My home. To sleep in my own bed.

It's as if my body is pulling me forward by a force attached to my left ring finger. The closer we get to home, the more nervous I feel. I haven't seen my husband in thirteen weeks. How will we act? How will we say hello? ? I feel like I've lived an entire lifetime since I last saw him. I'm not the same person as I was when I left. I have new scars, healed wounds, fresh ones. What scars did Jake develop while I was gone? Who is he after thirteen weeks without me?

Will Jake be able to understand what I've been through?

That's a stupid question. Of course he won't. No one could. The closest is Brad, and even he can't truly understand my experience, the same way I can't truly understand his. I haven't let myself miss Jake, miss home, miss Rieger. And now that I'm almost home, I miss them all so much that the thought of seeing them pierces straight through my heart. I have no idea how I'm going to convey my experiences, and the longing I feel, from head to toe, from my body to his ears.

A slight panic overtakes me when I emerged from the plane and don't see Jake. I rush to the baggage claim, but he isn't there, either. I walk towards the Southwest gates, searching the faces in the crowd for one that looks like his. Have I forgotten his features? Will I be able to recognize him from afar with a mask on? Has he gained weight? Lost it? Bought new clothes? What if he doesn't recognize me, either. My panic rises with each step, until finally I see a body across the walkway from me that is undoubtedly his. I pick up my pace to a sort of half-jog. I nearly run into a man who clearly isn't watching where he's going. I run the remaining ten feet to embrace Jake.

I hold onto his body as if my life depends on it. I haven't realized just how alone I've felt until I'm no longer alone. It's like, in the warmth of his embrace, I suddenly feel just how cold I have been, and in the moments we stand there together the cold seems as though it has been unsurvivable. It's like in the final few meters of a race, when you're nearly across the finish line, and only in those final few steps do you realize the absolute truth that you can barely take them, that you shouldn't have made it this far. But as you cross the finish line, you know that, in fact, you did. And you have absolutely no idea how.

Tears well my eyes, and I'm grateful for them, because I had feared I would lack emotion upon returning. I don't feel like I have any control over the way my body is currently attempting to regulate my various—and overwhelming—emotions. "I've missed you so much," I choke out, because it's all I can think to say. We grab my bags and make our way back to the car. Back to our apartment. Back to our lives.

That evening, we go to our friend's patio just as we have done a hundred nights before. So many of the people I love and cherish are there, together again. I listen quietly and contentedly as they yammer on about their lives since I left, just happy to be in their presence. In a moment between stories, I look up at the sky to breath in the night, and a shooting star passes by above my head. I smile and thank God that, in that moment, I have everything I could possibly ask for.

EPILOGUE

My anxieties will get the better of me several times over the next two weeks, but come the second week of August, I will receive an interview request from the original PACU job I wanted and a job offer for the one I interviewed with on my last day in New York. After much oscillation between the two jobs, I decide to accept both. I can faintly hear God telling me that *this* is how I will keep making money without traveling. *This* is how I will get rid of my car debt and student loans.

I spend the next three months working five days a week between the two jobs, sometimes including overnight shifts. It's hard, but if New York taught me anything, it's that I can do hard things. Since then, I have continued to chip away at my debts. I enjoy both jobs equally for different reasons, and I honestly couldn't choose one over the other. I feel very blessed to be able to say that; many people don't enjoy their *one* job.

On December 22, 2020, my boss came to me and said to check my email for a signup form to receive my first dose of the Pfizer vaccine. I couldn't believe it. I literally jumped up and down and squealed for joy. This was the best Christmas present I could possibly receive. *This* was what we had been hoping and praying for. *This* was the beginning of the road to relief from this horrific virus. I signed up to receive my first dose of the vaccine at the end of my shift alongside a couple of my work friends. Much to the dismay of the woman trying to corral me to the area where I would be receiving my own vaccine, I gleefully followed each friend to their booth to photograph them getting their shot, and then I took a selfie of myself getting mine. I was so happy looking around at all the people willing to go first, willing to do whatever was necessary to fight this virus, that I forgot to be afraid of the needle.

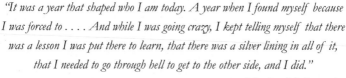

"It was a year that shaped who I am today. A year when I found myself because I was forced to . . . . And while I was going crazy, I kept telling myself that there was a lesson I was put there to learn, that there was a silver lining in all of it, that I needed to go through hell to get to the other side, and I did."

— *Matthew McConaughey*

"No one goes through hell and comes out the same on the other side."

— *Rachel Hollis*

ACKNOWLEDGEMENTS

To my dad. I wish you were here to read this, but I am thankful you did not have to live through the horrors of this pandemic. You were my favorite person, my hero. I miss you every day. All my love.

To my mom, who has suffered many of my spontaneous life choices, but who also raised me with the empowerment to make them in the first place. I love you.

To Elena. I truly believe that, if for no other reason, God called me to New York to meet you. You were exactly who I needed in this chapter of my life, and I am beyond grateful to have you by my side for the remaining chapters, even if it's from 1,200 miles away.

To Anna, my best friend. Our weekly FaceTime dates and your self-care birthday gift got me through this contract, and our weekly girl time now gets me through this messy thing called life. You have been there for me in ways no one else has, and I am so blessed to have a friend as amazing as you. Thank you for being my rock, even from 1,200 miles away.

To Kayla, my little sister (I know you're older than me, but I feel like I've corrupted you and that, therefore, I am the oldest). Your love and friendship have lasted longer than any other in my life. Thank you for always being by my side and having my back. For sending me love and chicken noodle soup from 1,200 miles away.

To my husband. Thank you for supporting my decision to go to New York. I missed you more than you could know those thirteen weeks we were apart. Thank you for your support while I was in Nursing School, and as I dealt with the gradual loss of my Dad. In many ways, you have helped shape who I am today.

To Hannah. I have no doubt that God spoke to me through you during our time together. I have not felt that with a friend in a long time. Please know that I pray for you and your family every day, and I cannot wait to run the NYC marathon with you.

To Ellie (not my dead dog, but my friend and fellow nurse). Your light and love for your patients and other people is infectious. You pushed me to be the best nurse I could be long after I stopped wanting to. Your positivity and smile got me through more shifts than I can count. Your laugh and your smile light up every room you walk into. Thanks for shining a little light into my life every day since we met.

To Liz. Thank you for being my work wife. There are many shifts I would not have survived without you, and a handful of Friday nights that I wouldn't have wanted to spend with anyone else.

To Lexi. Thank you for loving me. You saw many sides of me that I prefer to keep private, and you didn't judge me for them. There are a handful of shifts I wouldn't have survived without you. My patients probably wouldn't have survived them, either.

To Staci. I was beyond grateful to have a little piece of home nearby, and I feel so lucky to have gained such an amazing friend in the process.

To Lauren. You're the first girl I bonded with in New York, and I am so glad to have you as a friend. Thank you for being so welcoming, and for opening your home to me on more than one occasion while we were there. Congrats to you and Nicolai on your upcoming wedding!

To Carrie. Thanks for putting up with my diva moments. Thank you for the countless times you set up my CVVHD machines, and the endless help you offered not just me, but all the travel nurses. You are the reason I knew I would survive this contract.

To Anthony. Thank you for being one of the ICU nurses that just gets it. Thank you for all your help and kindness throughout my contract. P.S. I hope you're not cursed.

To Greg. Thanks for being a friend. A countless number of shifts were better because you were by my side. I will cherish my memories of your mutual love for dogs and your sailor scrub cap.

To Emily. There is no fellow (now MD—congrats lady!) I would have rather had by my side at the outbreak of a pandemic. All of my early memories of attempting to keep patients from coding have you in them. Thank you for being so amazing to work with.

To my favorite, pirate-hat-wearing, computer-skating, accented doctor (I hope you know who you are). Your desire to help others is infectious, and it was an honor to work by your side during my time in the ICU. And congratulations on your new baby girl.

To every single nurse I worked with in the ICU in Missouri. You were my family, and I feel very fortunate to have had such an amazing team to work with when we first began fighting this pandemic.

To all my parents' friends at Woods Chapel Church who sent me cards filled with words of encouragement throughout my contract. Those cards mean the world to me. I had them proudly displayed on top of the bookshelf in my room throughout my contract, and I display them in my home now to remind myself that no matter where I go, I am loved and well prayed for.

To George, thank you for being my number one cheerleader. Your support is everything. Falafel.

To Shawn, my editor. Thank you for helping me bring my story to life. Your encouragement in the fruition of this book has meant the world to me. Thank you for being its first reader, and for believing it is a story worth telling.

To JFM. Thank you for inspiring me to publish my writing, and for teaching me how to write better.

And finally, to you, my reader. Thank you for investing your time in my story. Any funds you invested in the purchase of this book will go towards paying off my nursing school student loan debt.

ABOUT THE AUTHOR

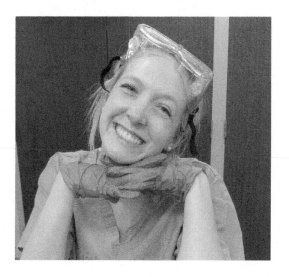

Laura Luther was born and raised an only child just outside of Kansas City, Missouri, where she now lives with her dog, Rieger. She earned her Bachelors in Science of Nursing with honors from the University of Missouri-Kansas City. Laura began her nursing career in the ICU at a trauma facility in Independence, Missouri. She now works as a pre-op nurse at a hospital in downtown Kansas City. During her four years as a nurse, Laura has received four different nominations for a DAISY Award. This memoir is her first published work as a writer.

Made in the USA
Coppell, TX
25 April 2022

77041397R00184